Ophthalmologic Drug Guide

Ophthalmologic Drug Guide
Second Edition

Douglas J. Rhee, MD
Associate Chief, Practice Development, Massachusetts Eye & Ear
Infirmary, Assistant Professor, Harvard Medical School, Boston,
Massachusetts, USA

Kathryn A. Colby, MD, PhD
Cornea Service, Massachusetts Eye & Ear Infirmary, Assistant
Professor, Harvard Medical School, Boston, Massachusetts, USA

Lucia Sobrin, MD, MPH
Assistant Professor, Harvard Medical School, Massachusetts Eye &
Ear Infirmary, Boston, Massachusetts, USA

Christopher J. Rapuano, MD
Director, Cornea Service, Wills Eye Hospital, Professor, Jefferson
Medical College, Philadelphia, Pennsylvania, USA

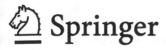 Springer

Douglas J. Rhee, MD
Harvard Medical School
Massachusetts Eye & Ear Infirmary
Boston, MA 02114, USA

Kathryn A. Colby, MD, PhD
Harvard Medical School
Massachusetts Eye & Ear Infirmary
Boston, MA 02114, USA

Lucia Sobrin, MD, MPH
Harvard Medical School
Massachusetts Eye & Ear Infirmary
Boston, MA 02114, USA

Christopher J. Rapuano, MD
Jefferson Medical College
Wills Eye Hospital
Philadelphia, PA 19107, USA

ISBN 978-1-4419-7620-8   e-ISBN 978-1-4419-7621-5
DOI 10.1007/978-1-4419-7621-5
Springer New York Dordrecht Heidelberg London

Printed on acid-free paper

Springer is part of Springer Science+Business Media (www.springer.com)

To my lovely wife Tina, for your continual patience and encouragement.
To my father and mother, Dennis and Serena Rhee, for your support and guidance.
To Susan Rhee for your understanding, and
To all my families – Rhee, Chang, Kim, and Chomakos.

Douglas J. Rhee

For Don, Amelia and Lilly, who fill my life with joy.

Kathryn A. Colby

To my supportive and loving husband, Jose, and my daughters, Carolina and Victoria, constant sources of laughter and joy.

Lucia Sobrin

To my wonderful wife and best friend, Sara, and to my wonderful children, Michael, Patrick, Daniel and Megan.
You keep me sane and constantly remind me of what is important in life.

Christopher J. Rapuano

Preface

This pocket reference is designed to assist the eye care professional by providing current information on the ever-increasing number of ocular pharmacotherapeutics. Many different classes of medications are listed, oftentimes with pertinent facts. This book presents the usual recommended dose for the medications listed. Clinical judgment should always be used, as all therapy should be tailored to the individual patient. The intent of this manual is to provide therapeutic suggestions once the diagnosis is known. We recommend its use in conjunction with an ophthalmologic reference text such as the *Massachusetts Eye & Ear Infirmary Illustrated Manual of Ophthalmology* (Saunders) or the *Wills Eye Manual: Office & Emergency Room Diagnosis and Treatment of Eye Disease* (Lippincott). A more complete listing of all mechanisms, side effects, and drug interactions can be found in the product insert, the *Physicians' Desk Reference*, and the *Physicians' Desk Reference for Ophthalmology*, and should be consulted.

Douglas J. Rhee, MD
Kathryn A. Colby, MD, PhD
Lucia Sobrin, MD, MPH
Christopher J. Rapuano, MD

Contents

List of Abbreviations

Abbreviations	Meaning
Dosing	
Qx	Every x hours
QOD	Every other day
QD	Once per day
BID	Twice per day
TID	Three times per day
QID	Four times per day
IV	Intravenous Administration
PO	Take by mouth
Weights and Measures	
mg	Milligram
Gm	Gram
kg	Kilogram
m^2	Meters mathematically squared (refers to body surface area)
ml	Milliliter
Formulation	
Soln	Solution
Susp	Suspension
Oint	Ointment
Tab	Tablet

1. Antibacterial Agents

D.J. Rhee et al., *Ophthalmologic Drug Guide*, 2nd ed.,
DOI 10.1007/978-1-4419-7621-5_1,
© Springer Science+Business Media, LLC 2011

A. TOPICAL ANTIBIOTICS*

Drug	Trade	Preparation	Dose	Notes
bacitracin	N/A	Soln, 10,000 u/ml	Q 1 hr	Fortified°
	AK-Tracin	Oint, 500 u/gm	QD-QID	BC
besifloxacin	Besivance	Suspension, 0.6%	TID-Q 1 hr	Fluoroquinolone-BC
cefazolin	Ancef	Soln, 5%	Q 1 hr	Fortified°
chloramphenicol	Chloromycetin, Chloroptic, Ocu-Chlor	Soln, 0.5%	Q 3–6 hrs	BS, except BC against *H. influenzae*, *N meningitidis*, *N. gonorrhea*, *C. trachomatis*. Has been reported to be associated with aplastic anemia.
	Chloromycetin, Chloroptic, Ocu-Chlor	Oint, 1%	QHS-Q 3 hrs	
ciprofloxacin	Ciloxan	Soln, 0.3%	QID-Q 1/2 hr	Fluoroquinolone-BC; active against *P. Aeruginosa* and *Neisseria* species
erythromycin	AK-mycin, Ilotycin	Oint, 0.3%	QHS-QID	BS; active against *N. gonorrhea* &
		Oint, 0.5%	QD-QID	*C. trachomatis*
gatifloxacin	Zymar	Soln, 0.3%	QID-Q1 hr	Fluoroquinolone-BC
	Zymaxid	Soln, 0.5%	QD-Q1 hr	
gentamicin	Garamycin, Genoptic, Gentacidin, Gentak, Ocu-mycin	Soln, 0.3%	Q 1–6 hrs	Aminoglycoside-BC; active against *P. Aeruginosa* and *N. gonorrhea*
	Garamycin, Genoptic, Gentacidin, Gentak, Ocu-mycin	Oint, 0.3%	QD-TID	
	N/A	Soln, 1.5%	Q 1 hr	Fortified°

levofloxacin	Quixin	Soln, 0.5%	QID-Q 1/2 hr	Fluoroquinolone-BC; active against *P. Aeruginosa* and *Neisseria* species
	Iquix	Soln, 1.5%	Q 30 1/2 hr-QID	
metronidazole	MetroGel	Gel, 0.75%	BID	Periocular use for rosacea **Not for use in the eye**
moxifloxacin	Vigamox	Soln, 0.5%	TID-Q1 hr	Fluoroquinolone-BC; Self Preserved; pH 6.8
neomycin	only available in combination medications (see below)			
norfloxacin	Chibroxin	Soln, 0.3%	QID-Q 1 hr	Fluoroquinolone- BC
ofloxacin	Ocuflox	Soln, 0.3%	QID-Q 1 hr	Fluoroquinolone- BC; active against *P. Aeruginosa* and *Neisseria* species;
oxytetracycline/ polymyxin B	AK-tetra, Terramycin, Terak	Oint, 0.5%/10,000 u	QD-QID	BC
polymyxin B/ bacitracin	AK-poly-bac, Polysporin, Polytracin	Oint, 10,000 u per ml/500 u per ml	QD-QID	BC
polymyxin B/ neomycin	AK-trol, Statrol	Soln, 16,250 u per ml/ 0.35%	QID	BC
	AK-trol, Statrol	Oint, 10,000 u per ml/ 0.35%	QD-QID	
polymyxin B/ neomycin/ bacitracin	Neotal	Oint, 5,000 u per ml/ 0.5%/ 400 u per ml	QD- QID	BC
	AK-spore, Neosporin, Ocu-spor B	Oint, 10,000 u per ml/ 0.35%/ 400 u	QD-QID	

(continued)

Antibacterial Agents 3

A. TOPICAL ANTIBIOTICS* *(continued)*

Drug	Trade	Preparation	Dose	Notes
polymyxin B/ neomycin/ gramicidin	AK-Spore, Neosporin, Ocu-spor G, Polymycin	Soln, 10,000 u per ml/ 0.35%/0.025%	QID	BC, gramicidin makes cell membrane more permeable
polymyxin B/ trimethoprim	Polytrim	Soln, 10,000 u per ml/ 0.1%	QID	BC
sulfacetamide	AK-sulf, Bleph-10, Ophthacet, Ocusulf, Sulf-10	Soln, 10%	QID-Q 1 hr	BS
sulfacetamide/ phenylephrine	AK-sulf Vasosulf	Oint, 10% Soln, 15%/0.125%	QD-QID QD-QID	BS; antibiotic with an alpha agonist
sulfisoxazole	Gantrisin Gantrisin	Soln, 4% Oint, 4%	QID-Q 1 hr QD-QID	BS
tetracycline	Achromycin	Soln, 1%	QID-Q 1/2 hr	BS
tobramycin	AKTOB, Defy, Tobrex	Soln, 0.3%	QID-Q 1 hr	Aminoglycoside – BC active against *P. Aeruginosa* and *N. gonorrhea*
	AKTOB, Defy, Tobrex	Oint, 0.3%	QD-TID	
vancomycin		Soln, 1.5%	Q 1 hr	Fortified◊
		Soln, 5%	Q 1 hr	BS, fortified◊, **not** for Gram negative coverage; reserve use for PCN allergic patients and resistant organisms

* For antibiotic spectrum of topical agents, refer to Appendix 1
◊ Fortified medications not commercially available; refer to Appendix 2 for preparation instructions
BC = bacteriocidal; BS = bacteriostatic; N/A = not available

B. ORAL ANTIBIOTICS

Drug	Trade	Dose	Notes
amoxicillin	Amoxil, Polymox	250–500 mg PO TID	Adult Dose
		25–50 mg/kg/day PO in 3 divided doses	Pediatric Dose
amoxicillin/clavulanate	Augmentin	250–500 mg PO TID or 875 mg PO BID	Adult Dose
		20–40 mg/kg/day PO in 3 divided doses	Pediatric Dose
azithromycin	Zithromax	500 mg PO day 1, then 250 mg QD × 4 days	Adult Dose
		20 mg/kg ×1 (pediatric dose)	Dose for *Chlamydia* conjunctivitis (Arch Ophthalmol 1998;116:1625–28 Ophthalmology 1998;105:658–61)
		1000 mg PO × 1 (adult dose)	
		5–12 mg/kg/day PO in one dose for 5 days	Pediatric Dose
cephalexin	Keflex	25–500 mg PO QID	Adult Dose
		25–50 mg/kg/day PO in 4 divided doses	Pediatric Dose
cefuroxime axetil	Ceftin	250–500 mg PO BID	Adult Dose
		20–30 mg/kg/day PO divided BID	Pediatric Dose
ciprofloxacin	Cipro	250–750 mg PO BID	Not for children or pregnancy Do not take with antacids must modify dosage in renal failure
	Cipro XE	500 mg PO QD	Extended release formula
clarithromycin	Biaxin	250–500 mg PO BID	Adult Dose
		15 mg/kg/day PO divided BID	Pediatric Dose

(continued)

B. ORAL ANTIBIOTICS *(continued)*

Drug	Trade	Dose	Notes
doxycycline	Vibramycin	100 mg BID	Can be used for ocular rosacea
erythromycin	E-mycin	250–500 mg PO QID 30–50 mg/kg/day in 3–4 divided doses	Not for children or pregnancy Adult Dose Pediatric Dose
gatifloxacin	Avelox	400 mg PO QD	Not for children or pregnancy
levofloxacin	Levaquin	500 mg PO QD	Not for children or pregnancy; must modify dosage in renal failure
minocycline	Minocin	100–200 mg PO BID	Not for children or pregnancy
moxifloxacin	Tequin	400 mg PO QD	Not for children or pregnancy
ofloxacin	generic	200–400 mg PO BID	Not for children or pregnancy; must modify dosage in renal failure
tetracycline	Achromycin	250–500 mg PO QID	Can be used for ocular rosacea Not for children or pregnancy Do not take with food, milk products, or antacids

C. ANTIBIOTICS FOR SUBCONJUNCTIVAL/INTRAVITREAL INJECTION

	Subconjunctival Injection*	Intravitreal Injection**	Notes
(1) Aminoglycosides$^\Psi$			
amikacin	25 mg	0.2–0.4 mg	
gentamicin	10–20 mg	0.2–0.4 mg	
kanamycin	30 mg	N/A	
neomycin	125–250 mg	N/A	rarely used
tobramycin	10–20 mg	0.1–0.4 mg	
(2) Penicillins			
ampicillin	50–150 mg	0.5 mg	rarely used
carbenicillin	100 mg	0.25–2.0 mg	
methicillin	50–100 mg	1.0–2.0 mg	
penicillin G	0.5–1.0 million units	N/A	
ticarcillin	100 mg	N/A	
(3) Cephalosporins			
cefazolin	100 mg	2.0–2.25 mg	1st Generation, rarely used
ceftazidime	200 mg	2.25 mg	3rd Generation

(continued)

C. ANTIBIOTICS FOR SUBCONJUNCTIVAL/INTRAVITREAL INJECTION (continued)

	Subconjunctival Injection[•]	Intravitreal Injection[••]	Notes
(4) Others			
bacitracin	5,000 units	N/A	
chloramphenicol	N/A	1.0 mg	rarely used
clindamycin	15–50 mg	1.0 mg	
erythromycin	100 mg	0.5 mg	
polymyxin B sulfate	100,000 units	N/A	almost never used
vancomycin	25 mg	1.0 mg	almost never used

[•] subconjunctival dose should be in a volume of 0.5 ml
[••] intravitreal dose should be in a volume of 0.1 ml
[Ψ] all intravitreal injections of aminoglycosides have potential for macular necrosis
N/A = not available

D. REGIMENS FOR SPECIFIC ORGANISMS

(1) Syphilis (caused by *Treponema Pallidum*) (*Expert Opin Pharmacother* 2005;6:2271)

Note: Both patient and sexual partners must be evaluated for other sexually transmitted diseases, including HIV.

(a) Early (Primary, secondary, or latent infection less than one year)

Drug	Dose
penicillin G benzathine	2.4 million U IM once (may repeat 7 days later in patients with AIDS)
OR	
one of the following for penicillin-allergic patients:	
doxycycline	100 mg PO BID × 14 days
azithromycin	2 Gm PO × 1
erythromycin	500 mg PO Q 6 hrs × 14 days

(b) Late (Includes isolated anterior uveitis; latent infection more than one year's duration; cardiovascular; gumma)

Drug	Dose
penicillin G benzathine	2.4 million U IM weekly × 3 weeks
or	
doxycycline	100 mg PO BID × 4 weeks

(c) Neurosyphilis (Includes posterior uveitic involvement)

Note: PCN allergic patients may need to be desensitized

Drug	Dose
penicillin G	2–4 million U IV Q 4 hrs × 10–14 days followed by penicillin G benzathine 2.4 MU IM Q week × 3

(d) Congenital

Drug	Dose
penicillin G	50,000 U/kg IM or IV Q 8–12 hrs × 10–14 days

(2) Gonococcal Conjunctivitis/Keratitis (caused by *Neisseria gonorrhea*) (*The Medical Letter*, 37:119, 1995)

Notes: 1) Patient's sexual partners must be treated. Both patient and sexual partners must be evaluated for other manifestations of gonorrhea and for other sexually transmitted diseases, including HIV and syphilis

2) Patients must also be treated for concurrent chlamydial infection, which may be present.

3) In penicillin/cephalosporin-allergic patients, consider ciprofloxacin 500 mg PO for one dose; an infectious disease consult may be needed.

4) All patients should receive warm saline irrigation of fornices
5) Also administer topical antibiotics:
- bacitracin or erythromycin ointment QID [may use ciprofloxacin, ofloxacin, gatifloxacin, or moxifloxacin soln Q 2 hrs (adults only)] for conjunctivitis only
- gatifloxacin, moxifloxacin, besifloxacin, ofloxacin, ciprofloxacin or gentamicin or tobramycin soln Q 1 hr for **corneal** involvement

Drug	Trade	Dose	Notes
ceftriaxone	Rocephin	1 gram IM × 1 dose	for adult GC conjunctivitis
		25–50 mg/kg IV QD × 7 days	for child with GC conjunctivitis[Λ]
		125 mg IM × 1 dose	for **Neonatal Gonococcal conjunctivitis**; do not use with hyperbilirubinemic neonates
cefotaxime	Claforan	1–2 gram IV QD × 3–5 days	for adult GC corneal ulcer
		50 mg/kg IV or IM Q 8–12 hrs × 7 days	for **Neonatal Gonococcal conjunctivitis**

(3) **Chlamydial Inclusion Conjunctivitis** (caused by *C. Trachomatis* Subtypes D-K)
   Trachoma (caused by *C. Trachomatis* Subtypes A, B, C)

Notes:

1) Duration of treatment is 3 weeks for inclusion conjunctivitis and 3–6 weeks for trachoma [Φ] . Oral azithromycin may be given as a single dose.
2) Diagnosis of inclusion conjunctivitis requires that patient's sexual partners be treated. Both patient and sexual partners must be evaluated for other sexually transmitted diseases, including HIV.
3) Select one ointment **and** one oral agent

Drug	Trade	Dose	Notes
erythromycin	AK-mycin, Ilotycin	Oint, 0.5% BID-TID × 3–6 weeks	recommended for **Neonatal Chlamydial** Conjunctivitis
oxytetracycline/polymyxin B	AK-tetra, Terramycin, Terak	Oint, 0.5%/10,000 u BID-TID × 3–6 weeks	Not for children or pregnancy
sulfacetamide	AK-sulf, Bleph-10, Cetamide, Sulamyd Sodium	Oint, 10% BID-ID × 3–6 weeks	
PLUS			
azithromycin	Zithromax	20 mg/kg ×1 (pediatric dose) 1000 mg PO × 1 (adult dose)	Effective as a single dose (Arch Ophthalmol 1998;116:1625–28 Ophthalmology 1998;105:658–61)
clarithromycin	Biaxin	250–500 mg PO BID for 3–6 weeks 15 mg/kg/day PO divided BID for 3–6 weeks	Adult Dose Pediatric Dose
doxycycline	Vibramycin	100 mg PO BID × 3–6 weeks	Not for children or pregnancy
erythromycin	E-mycin	250–500 mg PO QID × 3–6 weeks 50 mg/kg/day PO divided QID for 3–6 weeks	Adult Dose Pediatric Dose, recommended for 14 days in **Neonatal Chlamydial** Conjunctivitis
ofloxacin	Floxin	300 mg PO BID for 3–6 weeks	Not for children or pregnancy
tetracycline	Achromycin	250–500 mg PO QID × 3–6 weeks	Not for children or pregnancy

(4) Lyme Disease[Γ] (*Borrelia burgdorferi*): if patient has ocular involvement beyond follicular conjunctivitis occurring within the first month of infection, must be considered to have CNS involvement.

(a) Stage 1 (erythema migrans):

Early (limited to follicular conjunctivitis as above) select **one** agent and treat for 14 to 21 days (except azithromycin)[TB]:

Drug	Trade	Dose	Notes
amoxicillin	Amoxil	500 mg PO TID	Preferred first line agent
azithromycin	Zithromax	20–40 mg/kg/day PO in 3 divided doses	Pediatric Dose
		500 mg PO QD × 1 day, then	
		250 mg PO QD × 4 days	
cefuroxime	Ceftin	500 mg PO BID	Adult Dose
		20–30 mg/kg/day PO divided **BID**	Pediatric Dose (max 1 g QD)
clarithromycin	Biaxin	250–500 mg PO BID	Adult Dose
		15 mg/kg/day PO divided **BID**	Pediatric Dose
doxycycline	Vibramycin	100 mg PO BID	Preferred first line agent
			Not for children or pregnancy
erythromycin	E-mycin	250 mg PO QID	Adult Dose
		30–50 mg/kg/day in 3–4 divided doses	Pediatric Dose
tetracycline	Achromycin	250 mg PO QID	Not for children or pregnancy

(b) Stage 2

Develops in days to months with dissemination of organism to skin, heart, joints and CNS. Ocular involvement consists of granulomatous anterior uveitis, retinal vasculitis, choroiditis. Select **one** agent – patient needs systemic work-up to rule out arthritis, which must be treated with ceftriaxone or doxycycline

Drug	Trade	Dose	Notes
cefotaxime	Claforan	3 Gm IV Q 12 hrs × 21–28 days	Preferred first line agent
ceftriaxone	Rocephin	2.0 Gm IV QD × 21–28 days	Pediatric Dose (max 2 g/day)
		50–75 mg/kg/day divided Q 12 hrs	
doxycycline	Vibramycin	100 mg PO BID	Preferred first line agent
penicillin G		2–4 MU IV Q 4 hrs × 21–28 days	Not for children or pregnancy

(c) Stage 3

Develops weeks to years following initial infection and is typically characterized by development of arthritis. Ocular involvement includes episcleritis, stromal keratitis, orbital myositis.

Drug	Trade	Dose	Notes
ceftriaxone	Rocephin	2.0 gm IV QD × 14–28 days	Preferred first line agent
		50–75 mg/kg/day divided Q 12 hrs	Pediatric Dose (max 2 g/day)
or			
doxycycline	Vibramycin	100 mg PO BID × 30 days	Not for children or pregnancy

(5) Bartonella neuroretinitis (*Bartonella henselae, Bartonella quintana*)

Drug	Trade	Dose	Notes
rifampin and	Rifadin	300 mg PO BID × 4 weeks	LFTs should be monitored
doxycycline	Vibramycin	100 mg PO BID × 4 weeks	Not for children or pregnancy

ᴬ*Wills Eye Manual: Office and Emergency Room Diagnosis and Treatment of Eye Disease.*
ᶲCurrent Ocular Therapy 4. Fraunfelder, F., Roy, FH. 1995. Saunders Co. p. 62–63. [Current Ocular Therapy 6. Roy, FH, Fraunfelder, FW, Fraunfelder FT, Saunders Elsevier, 2008, p. 86–89.]
ᴦSanford Guide to Antimicrobial Therapy. Sanford, JP., Gilbert, DN., Sande, MA. 1995. p. 38–39.

E. REGIMENS FOR SPECIFIC CLINICAL ENTITIES

(1) Blepharitis

Notes:

1) Treated with combination of warm compresses, lid hygiene (using warm wash cloth with baby shampoo to scrub lashes), and artificial tears 4–8×/day depending on the severity of dry eye symptoms. Commercial lid scrub products also available, see below

2) May supplement with either erythromycin or bacitracin ointment at bedtime.

3) Additionally, may use a combination antibiotic/steroid (e.g. Vasocidin, Blephamide) QID. However, we recommend short duration of treatment and extreme care to monitor for side effects of topical steroids.

4) Cyclosporine 0.05% drops BID can be effective for posterior blepharitis, but often takes weeks-months to have a significant effect.

5) For severe posterior blepharitis or ocular rosacea, may supplement with an oral agent (see section on **rosacea, ocular**).

Drug	Trade	Dose	Notes
azithromycin	Azasite	bid × 2 days then qhs to eyes or lids	Off-label use
cocamindopropyl hydroxysultaine	OcuSoft Lid Scrub	scrub lids QD-QID	cocamindopropyl hydroxysultaine is a mild surfactant; preserved with quaternium-15
cocoamidopropylamide oxide	Lid Wipes	scrub lids QD-QID	
cyclosporine	Restasis	oil emulsion, 0.05% BID	Off label use, may take weeks to months to have a significant effect
	Novartis Eye Scrub OcuClenz	scrub lids QD-QID	

(2) Rosacea, Ocular

Select **one** agent, in addition to warm compresses, lid hygiene, and artificial tears. For oral agents, treat for 2–6 weels, then decrease dosing frequency by half (e.g. BID → QD) and continue for several months. After several months, the dose can be cut in half again in many patients.

Drug	Trade	Dose	Notes
azithromycin	Azasite	bid × 2 days then qhs to eyes or lids	Off-label use
doxycycline	Vibramycin	100 mg PO BID	Not for children or pregnancy
erythromycin	E-mycin	250 mg PO QID	If unable to take doxycycline or tetracycline
metronidazole	MetroGel	Gel, 0.75%, apply BID	Periocular use for rosacea **Not for use in the eye**
tetracycline	Achromycin	250 mg PO QID	Not for children or pregnancy
cyclosporin	Restasis	oil emulsion, 0.05% BID	Off-label use, may take weeks to months to have a significant effect

(3) Stye/Hordeolum

Notes:
1) Warm compress with massage over the affected area for 10–15 minutes four times per day.
2) Medications are not indicated unless **preseptal cellulitis** occurs (see subject index)
3) For **chalazion**, see Chapter X: Miscellaneous Conditions

(3.5) Chalazion/Hordeolum

Notes:
1) Warm compress with massage over the affected area four times per day.
2) If the lesion does not disappear after 3–4 weeks, then can consider surgical removal (incision and curettage) or steroid injection. Steroid injection can lead to permanent depigmentation of the skin at the injection site. If steroid injection is elected, can use 0.2–1.0 ml of a 40 mg/ml solution of triamcinolone (Kenalog).

(4) Pediculosis (*Phthirus pubis*, lice, "crabs")

Notes:
1) Use anti-lice lotion and shampoo for non-ocular areas: e.g. piperonyl butoxide/permethrins (e.g. Rid), permethrin (e.g. Elimite) or Lindane Shampoo.
2) Additionally, lice and nits (eggs) may be removed from lids/lashes with fine forceps at the slit lamp.
3) All sexual partners need to be examined; instruct the patient to wash and machine dry linens and sheets.
4) Physostigmine interferes with the organism's respiratory function, but has significant ocular side effects and is rarely used.

Drug	Trade	Dosage	Notes
Any bland ophthalmic ointment (bacitracin, erythromycin) to eyelids TID for 10 days (smothers lice and nits)			
OR			
physostigmine	Eserine	Oint, 0.25%	2 applications to lids 1 week apart; has significant ocular side effects; rarely used.

(5) Conjunctivitis

(a) Viral:

Anti-bacterial medications are not indicated in most viral conjunctivitis unless significant corneal epithelial damage has occurred to prevent secondary bacterial infections. For symptomatic improvement, consider artificial tears, ocular decongestant/antihistamine (i.e. naphazoline/pheniramine), topical nonsteroidals, and cool compresses.

(b) Bacterial:

If clinically suspect bacterial conjunctivitis, Gram stain and culture appropriately and start on a broad spectrum topical agent (e.g. azithromycin 1–2 × day, polymyxin/trimethoprim, ciprofloxacin, ofloxacin, levofloxacin 4–8 ×/day or gatifloxacin, moxifloxacin, besifloxacin 3–6 ×/day). Certain etiologies (i.e. *Neisseria gonorrhea*) are relative emergencies and should be managed according to specific regimens.

(c) Neonatal:

Most commonly caused by *Chlamydia trachomatis, Strep. viridans, Staph. aureus, Haemophilus influenzae,* group B *Streptococcus, Moraxella catarrhalis, or Neisseria gonorrhea.* Treatment is guided by gram stain (which should be performed immediately to identify *N. gonorrhea* and *C. trachomatis* have specific regimens as described (see Neonatal Gonococcal Conjunctivitis and Neonatal Chlamydial Conjunctivitis in subject index). If not gonococcal or chlamydial, may use erythromycin or bacitracin ointment Q 4–6 hrs. as only initial treatment. In the United States, neonatal conjunctivits is most commonly chlamydial.

(6) Canaliculitis

Notes: 1) Etiologies include *Actinomyces Israelii* (most common), viruses, chlamydia, fungi, and other bacteria.
2) Surgical removal of offending agent is the most important aspect of treatment. Evaluate drainage system for obstruction, attempt to remove concretions, and obtain smears and cultures of any material expressed.

3) Consider irrigation of canaliculus with penicillin G solution 100,000 units/ml, repeat as necessary; irrigation should be performed in upright position so drainage is out nose rather than nasopharynx.

4) Consider tetracycline 250 mg PO QID (not for use in children or pregnancy) or Bactrim DS 1 tab PO BID, for bacterial etiologies.

5) If fungus is recovered, irrigate with nystatin 1:20,000 units/ml in addition to topical nystatin drops TID.

6) If herpes is found, treat with trifluridine 1% drops 5×/day for several weeks.

7) Warm compresses QID.

8) Canaliculotomy may be necessary to prevent recurrent infections due to the tendency for diverticuli formation that may harbor concretions and additional organisms

(7) Dacryocystitis

Notes:

1) All patients receive topical polymyxin/trimethoprim (Polytrim) QID in addition to systemic antibiotics

2) All patients receive warm compresses QID

3) May require surgical incision & drainage if abscess is present

4) May require surgical reconstruction of nasolacrimal drainage system (e.g. DCR) 1–4 weeks after acute inflammation is resolved

5) Fungal etiologies usually have a more subacute or chronic presentation; aspergillus is most common fungal cause (see **Aspergillosis**)

6) Pediatric consultation is recommended in children

7) Recent studies suggest an increase in methicillin-resistant Staphylococcus aureus and gram negative pathogens as causative agents in dacrocystitis. Many affected patients harbor multiple organisms. This should be taken consider if clinical response to first-line agents is not as expected.

(a) Afebrile, mild case, systemically well, reliable patient/parent

Select **one** agent with daily follow-up

Drug	Trade	Dose	Notes
amoxicillin/clavulanate	Augmentin	500 mg PO TID or 875 mg PO BID	Adult Dose
		20–40 mg/kg/day PO in 3 divided doses	Pediatric Dose
cefaclor	Ceclor	250 mg PO TID	Adult Dose
		20–40 mg/kg/day PO in 3 divided doses	Pediatric Dose
cephalexin	Keflex	500 mg PO QID	Adult Dose
		25–50 mg/kg/day PO in 4 divided doses	Pediatric Dose

(b) Febrile, moderate-severe case, acutely ill, unreliable parent

Hospitalize and select **one** agent

Drug	Trade	Dose	Notes
cefazolin	Ancef	1 Gm IV Q 8 hrs	Adult Dose
		25–50 mg/kg/day IV in 3 divided doses	Pediatric Dose
cefuroxime	Zinacef	1.5 Gm IV Q 8 hrs	Adult Dose
		75–100 mg/kg/day IV in 3 divided doses	Pediatric Dose

(8) Dacryoadenitis—Bacterial

Notes:
1) Other causes of lacrimal gland masses include inflammatory, neoplastic, and viral causes. Please refer to the Wills Eye Manual: Office and Emergency Room Diagnosis and Treatment of Eye Disease for complete discussion on evaluation of non-bacterial treatment.
2) CT scan of orbit and brain to rule out abscess formation which may require surgical incision & drainage
3) Pediatric consultation is recommended in children

(a) Mild

Select **one** agent with daily follow-up

Drug	Trade	Dose	Notes
amoxicillin/clavulanate	Augmentin	250–500 mg PO TID or 875 mg PO BID	Adult Dose
		20–40 mg/kg/day in 3 divided doses	Pediatric Dose
cephalexin	Keflex	250–500 mg PO QID	Adult Dose
		25–50 mg/kg/day in 4 divided doses	Pediatric Dose

(b) Moderate to Severe

Hospitalize and select **one** agent

Drug	Trade	Dose	Notes
ticarcillin/clavulanate	Timentin	3.1 Gm IV Q 4–6 hrs	Adult Dose
		200 mg/kg/day in 4 divided doses	Pediatric Dose above age 12
cefazolin	Ancef	1 Gm IV Q 8 hrs	Adult Dose
		50–100 mg/kg/day IV in 3 divided doses	Pediatric Dose over one month of age (max adult dose 4–6 g/day)

(9) Preseptal Cellulitis

(a) Mild case, patient > 5 years of age, afebrile, systemically well, reliable patient/parent

Select **one** agent with daily follow-up and treat for 10 days

Drug	Trade	Dose	Notes
amoxicillin/ clavulanate	Augmentin	250–500 mg PO TID or 875 PO BID	Adult Dose
		20–40 mg/kg/day PO in 3 divided doses	Pediatric Dose
cefaclor	Ceclor	250–500 mg PO TID	Adult Dose
		20–40 mg/kg/day PO in 3 divided doses	Pediatric Dose
cephalexin	Keflex	250–500 mg PO QID	Adult Dose
		25–50 mg/kg/day in 4 divided doses	Pediatric Dose
clarithromycin	Biaxin	250–500 mg PO BID	Adult Dose
		15 mg/kg/day PO divided BID	Pediatric Dose
erythromycin	E-mycin	250–500 mg PO QID	Adult Dose
		30–50 mg/kg/day PO in 3–4 divided doses	Pediatric Dose
			Not very good against Staphylococcus or Streptococcus
trimethoprim/ sulfamethoxazole	Bactrim	1 double strength tablet PO BID	Adult Dose
		8–12 mg/kg/day TMX & 40–60 mg/kg/day SMX PO in 2 divided doses	Pediatric Dose

(b) Moderate-Severe Preseptal Cellulitis or Child <5 years of age

Hospitalize and give **BOTH** agents

Drug	Trade	Dose	Notes
ceftriaxone	Rocephin	1–2 Gm IV Q 12 hrs	Adult Dose
		100 mg/kg/day IV in 2 divided doses	Pediatric Dose
AND			
vancomycin	Vancocin	0.5–1 GM IV Q 12 hrs	Adult Dose[Y]
		40 mg/kg/day IV in 3–4 divided doses	Pediatric Dose[Y]
		15 mg/kg load, maintenance dose 10 mg/kg BID-TID	Neonatal Dose[Y]

Notes:

1) Patient may be switched to oral therapy after significant improvement has occurred; total duration of systemic therapy should be for 10–14 days.
2) Children under 5 years must receive complete physical examination to rule out concurrent otitis media, sinusitis, and bacteremia. Pediatric consultation is recommended.
3) Widespread introduction of the Hemophilus influenza type B vaccine have reduced the frequency of preseptal cellulitis caused by this agent

[Y]Follow peak and trough levels; dosage must be adjusted in renal failure

(10) Orbital Cellulitis–Bacterial

(a) Children:

Give **BOTH** agents; pediatric consultation is recommended.

Drug	Trade	Dose	Notes
ceftriaxone	Rocephin	100 mg/kg/day IV in 2 divided doses	
AND			
vancomycin	Vancocin	40 mg/kg/day IV in 3–4 divided doses	Pediatric Dose[Y]
		15 mg/kg load, maintenance dose 10 mg/kg BID-TID	Neonatal Dose

(b) Adults:

Give either ampicillin/sulbactam alone or ceftriaxone plus vancomycin

Drug	Trade	Dose	Notes
ampicillin/sulbactam	Unasyn	1.5 Gm–3.0 Gm IV Q 6 hrs × 7 days	
ceftriaxone	Rocephin	1–2 Gm IV Q 12 hrs × 7 days	Continue oral antibiotics on discharge
vancomycin	Vancocin	1 Gm IV Q 12 hrs × 7 days[Y]	Continue oral antibiotics on discharge

Notes:

1) If highly suspect adults with anaerobic infections consider adding metronidazole 15 mg/kg IV load, then 7.5 mg/kg IV Q 6 hrs, or clindamycin 600 mg IV Q 8 hrs. (Ampicillin/sulbactam alone has adequate anaerobic coverage)

[Y]Follow peak and trough levels; dosage must be adjusted in renal failure

2) If adult patient is allergic to penicillin/cephalosporin, may use vancomycin plus gentamicin 2.0 mg/kg IV loading dose, then 1 mg/kg IV Q 8 hrs **or** clindamycin 600 mg IV Q 8 hrs plus gentamicin

3) Case reports have documented the appearance of methicillin-resistant Staphyloccus aureus as a causative agent in non-hospitalized adults and children.

4) Recent studies suggest that anaerobic bacteria may play a larger role in orbital cellultitis than previously thought. Consideration should be given to adding intravenous metronidazole (Flagyl; 7.5 mg/kg three times daily, max dose 400 mg), especially if the clinical exam does not improve with standard antibiotic therapy.

5) If no improvement, suspect abscess or resistant organism

6) Initial work-up should include orbital/sinus CT with contrast.

7) Children tend to do better on IV antibiotics than adults because they are less likely to have polymicrobial infections.

8) Adults often have a mix of anaerobes in addition to the usual infections agents, which may limit response to systemic antibiotics alone. Consider urgent surgical drainage for adults with subperiosteal abscesses.

9) Consider ENT evaluation for all patients with suspected sinus etiology.

(11) Prophylaxis of post-traumatic endophthalmitis following open globe injuries (including full thickness corneal laceration)

Notes:

1) On presentation shield eye without contact to globe and keep patient NPO.

2) Treatment is prompt surgical exploration and repair.

3) Admit and give systemic antibiotics for 36 hours – give **two** (i.e. vancomycin plus ceftazidime or vancomycin plus levofloxacin):

Drug	Trade	Dose	Notes
vancomycin	Vancocin	1 Gm IV Q 12 hrs 40 mg/kg/day IV in 2–4 divided doses 15 mg/kg load, maintenance dose 10 mg/kg BID-TID	Adult Dose[Y] Pediatric Dose[Y] Neonatal Dose[Y]
PLUS ceftazidime	Fortaz	1 Gm IV Q 8 hrs 25–50 mg/kg IV Q 8 hrs (max 6 g/day)	Adult Dose Pediatric Dose
OR levofloxacin	Levaquin	500 mg IV or po Q 24 hrs	Not approved for use in children Modify dose in renal failure
If vancomycin allergy consider: clindamycin	Cleocin	10–15 mg/kg IV or IM Q 6–12 hours	true allergy to vancomycin is uncommon

4) CT scan to rule out intraocular and/or intraorbital foreign body
5) Vancomycin should be infused slowly (over 1–2 hours) to prevent "red man" syndrome
5) If no endophthalmitis develops after 48–72 hours of IV therapy, may discontinue. If high risk for endophthalmitis (delayed presentation or intraocular foreign body, consider oral levoquin (500 mg daily for 1 week)
6) If tetanus immunization not up to date, give tetanus toxoid 0.5 ml IM.
7) If endophthalmitis does develop, see **endophthalmitis – traumatic**

Note: oral levofloxacin and moxifloxacin achieve good aqueous and vitreous penetration (**Ophthalmology** 1999;106:2286–2290; Am J Ophthalmol 2007;143:338–40) and can be used for completion of the antibiotic course in outpatient setting.

Antibacterial Agents 25

[Y] Follow peak and trough levels; dosage must be adjusted in renal failure

(12) Blebitis (most commonly associated with *Streptococcus* species and *Haemophilus influenzae*)

*(a) Suspected bleb infection but **NO** anterior chamber or vitreal involvement*

Notes:

1) Consider culturing bleb for diagnostic purposes
2) Select antibiotic regimen (use gatifloxacin or moxifloxacin alone or both fortified tobramycin and vancomycin)

Name	Trade	Preparation	Dose	Notes
gatifloxacin	Zymar	Soln, 0.3%	Q 1 hr	mild case
moxifloxacin	Vigamox	Soln, 0.5%	Q 1 hr	mild case
OR				
tobramycin (fortified)◇	Tobrex	Soln, 1.5%	Q 1 hr	moderate-severe case
and				
vancomycin (fortified)◇	Vancocin	Soln, 5%	Q 1 hr	moderate-severe case

3) In adults, consider oral ciprofloxacin 250–500 mg PO BID for 10 days; may also consider oral fourth generation fluor-oquinolone as well.
4) Re-evaluate after 12–24 hrs and if there is improvement consider adding steroid to prevent loss of bleb.

prednisolone acetate	Pred Forte, Econopred plus Susp,	1%	QID

*(b) Suspected bleb infection with anterior chamber but **NO** vitreal involvement*

Notes:

1) Consider culturing bleb and/or performing anterior chamber tap for diagnostic purposes.
2) Begin antibiotics immediately; use both drops alternating every half hour; consider admission to hospital.
3) In adults, consider oral ciprofloxacin 250–500 mg PO BID for 10 days; may also consider oral fourth generation fluor-oquinolone as well.

Name	Trade	Preparation	Dose	Notes
tobramycin (fortified)◊	Tobrex	Soln, 1.5%	Q 1 hr	
and				
cefazolin (fortified)◊	Ancef	Soln, 5%	Q 1 hr	
or				
vancomycin (fortified)◊	Vancocin	Soln, 5%	Q 1 hr	should be reserved for PCN allergic patients or resistant organisms

Note: 4) Re-evaluate after 12–24 hrs; if there is improvement, consider adding steroid to prevent loss of bleb.

prednisolone acetate   Pred Forte, Econopred Plus Susp,   1% Q 2 hr

(c) with anterior chamber and vitreal involvement – see endophthalmitis (see below)

(13) Endophthalmitis

(a) Postoperative-Acute (less than one week)

Most common organism encountered is *Staph. epidermidis*, others include *Staph. aureus*, *Streptococcus* species, *Serratia marcescens*, *Proteus* species, and *Pseudomonas* species

Notes:
1) Intravitreal antibiotics are the treatment of choice, combined with topical antibiotics; the benefit of subconjunctival antibiotics is unclear and is not frequently used.
2) Immediate pars plana vitrectomy is beneficial if visual acuity on presentation is light perception or worse (Arch Ophthalmol. 1995;113:1479–1496).
3) Often combined with topical, subconjunctival, and/or intravitreal steroids since fungi are unlikely in the early post-operative setting. Use topical prednisolone acetate 1% Q 1 hr and subconjunctival triamcinolone 40 mg at the time of vitrectomy. Intravitreal dexamethasone 0.4 mg at time of surgery is at surgeon's discretion. Some have shown that concomitant use of intravitreal steroids may yield a worse visual prognosis (Ophthalmology 2000;107:486–489).
4) Topical atropine 1% TID is also given for cycloplegia.

(1) Topical: combination of fortified aminoglycoside with either fortifed cefazolin or vancomycin

Drug	Dose
fortified cefazolin° OR fortified vancomycin°	Q 1 hr (alternate drops every 30 minutes)
PLUS	
fortified gentamicin° OR fortified tobramycin°	Q 1 hr (alternate drops every 30 minutes)

(2) Intravitreal: can be re-injected if the vitreous is not clearing

Note: Ceftazidime is alternative agent for Gram-negative coverage in bacterial endophthalmitis (Surv Ophthalmol. 41:395–401, 1997)

Drug	Dose
amikacin	0.2–0.4 mg in 0.1 ml
OR	
ceftazidime	2.25 mg in 0.1 ml
PLUS	
vancomycin	1.0 mg in 0.1 ml (clindamycin 1 mg in 0.1 ml may be used in place of vancomycin)

(3) Subconjunctival

Drug	Dose
ceftazidime	100 mg in 0.5 ml
AND	
vancomycin	25–50 mg in 0.5 ml

(b) Postoperative—Delayed (longer than one week)

Notes:

1) Begin treatment as with Postoperative-Acute except do **NOT** use steroids if fungal etiology is suspected.

2) Immediate pars plana vitrectomy is beneficial if visual acuity on presentation is light perception or worse up to six weeks following surgery (Arch Ophthalmol. 1995;113:1479–1496). Benefit beyond six weeks is not known.

3) If *Propionibacterium acnes* infection is suspected [usually from 2 months to several years following cataract surgery with granulomatous keratic precipitates, anterior uveitis, vitritis, and white plaques in capsular bag (often with retained lens material)], intravitreal vancomycin combined with local debridement/removal of intracapsular plaques may be sufficient.

4) If mild *Staph epidermidis* is isolated, intraocular vancomycin alone may be sufficient.

5) If fungus is suspected (usually begins approximately 3 months after surgery — *Candida* is most commonly encountered organism), consider amphotericin B 5–10 μg at time of vitrectomy. Amphotericin B has been reported to have retinal toxicity in animal studies. Therefore, if air-fluid exchange is performed for concurrent retinal detachment, the dose of amphotericin should be reduced by a third to one half.

6) If fungus is identified on Gram stain, Giemsa, or Calcofluor white, then use combination of topical and systemic antifungal medications. Natamycin 5% Q 1 hr is a good topical option. The antibiotic of choice for broad-spectrum systemic coverage has traditionally been Amphotericin B administered intravenously. Fluconazole 400–800 mg PO QD is also commonly used if the strain is sensitive. For fluconazole-resistant fungi, Voriconazole administered orally or intravenously at 200 mg twice daily can be used (Am J Ophthalmol 2005;139:135–140).

(c) Traumatic

Notes:

1) Begin treatment as with Postoperative-Acute except do **NOT** use steroids and therapeutic benefit of pars plana vitrectomy (PPV) is unknown for this type of endophthalmitis. However PPV offers the benefit of reducing infectious load and providing sufficient material for diagnostic culture and pathology.

2) Intravitreal amikacin 0.4 mg in 0.1 ml or ceftazidime 2.25 in 0.1 ml along with intravitreal vancomycin 1.0 mg in 0.1 ml should be given. May repeat Q 2–3 days. (clindamycin 1 mg in 0.1 ml may be used instead of vancomycin).

3) If wound or sclera is involved, consider addition of oral ciprofloxacin 250–750 mg BID.

4) Consider obtaining CT scan to rule out intraocular foreign body.

5) If tetanus immunization not up to date, give tetanus toxoid 0.5 ml IM.

6) Steroids should NOT be used until fungal organisms are ruled out. If no fungi are isolated, may use prednisolone acetate 1% Q 4 hrs and subconjunctival dexamethasone 4 mg. Prednisone 40–80 mg PO QD is at the discretion of the surgeon. If fungus is isolated, specific anti-fungal regimens may be used.

7) Incidence of post-traumatic endophthalmitis higher in rural settings; most common agents are *Staph. epidermidis, Bacillus* species, *Streptococcus* species, *Staph. aureus,* and various fungi.

(d) Endogenous—therapy is variable and treatment depends on suspected source

Notes:

1) Thorough physical examination must be performed to locate potential source of infection and consultation with an infectious disease specialist is desirable.

2) Broad spectrum IV antibiotics are used according to the suspected source of septic infection and blood culture results. IV drug users should receive aminoglycosides and clindamycin to eliminate possible *Bacillus cereus,* and vancomycin should be considered for *Staph. aureus* coverage. Other common associated pathogens include *Streptococcus* species and *Staph. aureus* with endocarditis, and *Candida* with indwelling catheters, hyperalimentation, and IV drug users.

3) Intravitreal antibiotics offer higher intraocular concentrations.

4) Vitrectomy offers the benefit of reducing infective load and providing sufficient material for diagnostic culture and pathology.

5) For fungal etiologies (see subject index for specific organisms), the decision to perform vitrectomy should be made when there is an inadequate response to systemic medications or advanced vitreous opacification on presentation.

ᵧ Follow peak and trough levels; dosage must be adjusted in renal failure

° Fortified medications not commercially available; refer to Appendix 2 for preparation instructions

2. Antifungal Agents[Π]

[Π]Refer to Appendix 3 for activity spectrum of anti-fungal agents

D.J. Rhee et al., *Ophthalmologic Drug Guide*, 2nd ed.,
DOI 10.1007/978-1-4419-7621-5_2,
© Springer Science+Business Media, LLC 2011

A. AGENTS

Drug	Trade	Concentration/Route of Admin.	Usual Dose	Notes
amphotericin B[Ω]	Fungizone	Soln, 0.15% Subconj Intravitreal IV	Q 1–6 hrs 0.8–1.0 mg 5 µg/0.1 ml 0.8–1.0 mg/kg/day	Varies depending on pathogen
fluconazole[Ωβ]	Diflucan	PO/IV	400 mg on day 1, then 100–400 mg QD	Max daily dose 400 mg
flucytosine[Ω]	Ancobon	Soln, 1% PO	Q 1–6 hrs 50–150 mg/kg in 4 divided doses	Varies depending on pathogen Used only as adjunctive treatment; serum levels must be followed
itraconazole[β]	Sporanox	PO	200 mg QD–BID	
ketoconazole[Ωβ]	Nizoral	PO	200–400 mg QD	Take with food
miconazole	Monistat	Soln, 1, 2% Subconj Intravitreal	Q 1–6 hrs 5–10 mg 10 µg	Varies depending on pathogen
natamycin	Natacyn	Susp, 5%	Q 1–6 hrs	Varies depending on pathogen
voriconazole	Vfend	200 mg Soln, 1% Intravitreal	PO BID Q 1–6 hrs 50 µg/0.1 ml	Varies depending on pathogen

[Ω]Toxic agent with potential severe side effects – refer to product information and warnings before use. Some side effects listed above.
[β]Drug has potential to interact with some medications and may precipitate acute ventricular arrythmia (i.e. terfenadine, astemizole, cisapride, triazolam).

Side Effects:

Drug	Preparation	Side Effects
amphotericin B[Ω]	Soln:	burning, irritation
	Subconj:	local ischemic necrosis, subconjunctival nodule
	Intravitreal:	chemosis, corneal clouding, possible risk of retinal toxicity
	Intravenous:	we recommend giving in consultation with infectious disease specialist or physician familiar with its use (consider a test dose to monitor for severe reaction). Rapid infusion can result in hypotension, hypokalemia, arrhythmias, and shock. Fever, chills, hypotension, and dyspnea are common. Nephrotoxicity, renal tubular acidosis, electrolyte abnormalities (hypokalemia and hypomagnesemia), anemia, headache, nausea, vomiting, malaise, weightloss, phlebitis, thrombocytopenia, mild leukopenia.
fluconazole[Ωβ]	PO:	GI distress, allergic rash, eosinophillia, Stevens-Johnson syndrome, transaminase elevation, thrombocytopenia. Increases concentrations of phenytoin, sulfonylureas, warfarin, and cyclosporine.
flucytosine[Ω]	Soln:	burning, irritation (typically less than amphotericin)
	PO:	marrow suppression leading to leukopenia and thrombocytopenia, rash, nausea, vomiting, severe enterocolitis, hepatotoxicity, renal toxicity, and cardiac arrest.
itraconazole[β]	PO:	nausea, vomiting, rash, pruritus, weakness, dizziness, vertigo, pedal edema, paresthesias, impotence, loss of libido.
ketoconazole[Ωβ]	PO:	nausea, anorexia, vomiting, allergic rash, pruritus, gynecomastia, decreased libido/impotence, hypertension, and fluid retention secondary to concentrations of adrenalcortical steroids, elevated LFTs
miconazole	Soln:	burning, itching, irritation
	Subconj:	generally well tolerated
natamycin	Soln:	less irritating than amphotericin
voriconazole	PO:	visual disturbances, fever, rash, vomiting, nausea, diarrhea, headache transaminase elevation, need to monitor liver function tests
	Soln:	burning, irritation

[Ω]Toxic agent with potential severe side effects – refer to product information and warnings before use. Some side effects listed above.
[β]Drug has potential to interact with some medications and may precipitate acute ventricular arrythmia (i.e. terfenadine, astemizole, cisapride, triazolam).

Antifungal Agents   33

B. SPECIFIC ANTI-FUNGAL REGIMENS

Special Note on Fungal Keratitis: Although the regimens are given for specific organisms, the major differentiation is between ulcers caused by yeast—for which amphotericin B is the drug of choice—or mold (most commonly *Fusarium*)—for which natamycin is generally the preferred agent. Voriconazole is also often effective for yeasts and molds. Mechanical debridement of superficial lesions removes necrotic tissue and may aid with antifungal medication penetration. Therapeutic penetrating keratoplasty should be considered for progressive disease or deep penetration to prevent development of endophthalmitis.

(1) Yeast

(a) Candidiasis (*Candida albicans*)

Candida albicans involvement of eye beyond eyelid skin and conjunctivitis is usually part of systemic involvement; therefore, a systemic evaluation is needed.

Notes: 1) *Eyelid skin or conjunctival involvement:* fluconazole 400 mg PO QD with food

2) *Keratitis*[δ]: Topical amphotericin B drops Q 1/2–1 hr occasionally with either oral voriconazole, ketoconazole, itraconazole, or fluconazole. If no improvement, consider PKP. Some advocate addition of flucytosine drops Q 1/2 – 1 hr (Int. Ophthalmol. Clinics Summer 1996; vol 36 (3):1–15) or voriconazole 1% drops Q 1 hr.

3) *Retinitis/Uveitis/Endophthalmitis*[φ]: fluconazole 400–800 mg PO QD for 4–6 weeks. In resistant cases, may substitute with intravenous amphotericin B 1 mg/kg/day for total dose of 2 gms or Voriconazole 200 mg PO BID. Intravitreal amphotericin B 5 µg at time of vitrectomy may also be given. There are reports of successful use of intravitreal voriconazole (100 µg/0.1 mL) in Candidal endophthalmitis (Am J Ophthalmol 2005;139:135). If source is traumatic inoculation, refer to **endophthalmitis – traumatic** in the subject index. If source is endogenous, refer to **endophthalmitis – endogenous** in the subject index.

(b) Cryptococcus (Cryptococcus neoformans)

Must rule out CNS involvement and underlying immunosuppression or AIDS because **meningitis** is treated differently.

Notes: 1) *Keratitis*[δ]: Topical amphotericin B drops Q 1/2–1 hr. with either oral voriconazole, fluconazole, ketoconazole, or itraconazole. If no improvement consider PKP. Some advocate addition of flucytosine drops Q 1/2–1 hr (Int. Ophthalmol. Clinics Summer 1996; vol 36 (3):1–15) or voriconazole Q 1hr

2) *Choroiditis*[Φ]: If isolated choroiditis, then use amphotericin B 0.5–0.8 mg/kg/day with flucytosine 2 Gm PO Q 6 hrs × 8–10 weeks (Retina. 10: 27–32. 1990); if unresponsive or endophthalmitis/significant vitritis develops, may use intravitreal amphotericin B with vitrectomy (Retina. 7: 75–79, 1987)

(2) Molds

(a) Aspergillosis (Aspergillus) (filamentous fungus, septate hyphae)

Notes: 1) *Dacryocystitis:* Surgical removal of 'aspergilloma' with possible surgical reconstruction of nasolacrimal drainage system is the definitive treatment. Antifungal medication is not generally required.

2) *Keratitis*[δ]: First choice is topical amphotericin B drops Q 1 hr initially with oral voriconazole, ketoconazole or fluconazole; Second choice topical agent is voriconazole or natamycin.Consider miconazole drops for infections refractory to amphotericin B, voriconazole, and natamycin.

3) *Endophthalmitis*[Φ]: Intravitreal and subconjunctival amphotericin B with vitrectomy. Should evaluate for systemic involvement. There are isolated reports of successful use of voriconazole (100 μg/0.1 mL) in Aspergillus endophthalmitis (Ophthalmology 2006;113:1184).

4) *Orbital infection*[Φ]: Requires surgical debridement with intravenous amphotericin B.

(b) Fusarium (filamentous fungus, septate hyphae)

Notes: 1) *Keratitis*[δ]: First choice topical agent is natamycin every 30 min to 1 hr for first two days; second line topical agents are voriconazole, miconazole, or flucytosine.

(c) Mucormycosis[φ] *(Zygomycosis) (filamentous fungus, nonseptate hyphae)*

Notes: 1) *Keratitis*[δ]/*Endophthalmitis*[φ]: Due to the highly invasive nature, would recommend local treatment with topical amphotericin B and systemic amphotericin B. Consider surgical debridement.

2) *Orbital infection*[φ]: Use intravenous amphotericin B; may require surgical debridement with topical amphotericin B washings.

(3) Dimorphic Fungi

(a) Blastomycosis[φ] *(Blastomyces dermatitidis)*

Notes: 1) *Granulomatous Blepharoconjunctivitis*: Itraconazole 200 mg PO QD or voriconazole 200 mg PO BID × 6 months. All extrapulmonary blastomycosis needs to be treated systemically. With severely ill patients, consider systemic amphotericin B.

2) *Keratitis*[δ]: As above with addition of topical voriconazole or miconazole drops.

(b) Coccidioidomycosis[φ] *(Coccidioides immitis)*

Note: May get phlyctenular conjunctivitis, episcleritis, or scleritis as part of symptomatic primary infection syndrome "Valley Fever". These are self limited and do not require treatment since they are felt to be a hypersensitivity reaction to coccidiodal antigens.

1) *Posterior Uveitis*: Many times, involvement is asymptomatic and resolve spontaneously. Symptomatic involvement (e.g. chronic granulomatous iridocyclitis, choroiditis, and retinitis) is usually associated with progressive systemic coccidiomycosis. Life threatening disease, such as meningeal involvement, is treated with IV amphotericin B. Non life threatening disease may be treated with fluconazole 400–600 mg PO QD × 9–12 months or voriconazole 200 mg PO BID × 9–12 months, or itraconazole 200 mg PO BID × 12 months.

(c) *Histoplasmosis (Histoplasma capsulatum)*

Note: 1) *Choroiditis:* Typically not treated by medications. However, patients must be monitored for choroidal neovascularization which may require laser, photodynamic, or intravitreal anti-angiogensis therapy.

(d) *Sporotrichosis*[φ] *(Sporothrix schenckii)*

Notes: 1) *Eyelid skin:* Preferred drug is itraconazole 200 mg PO BID. Alternatively, may use 10 drops of saturated potassium iodide PO TID; increase until total daily dose of 120 drops. Consider concurrent use of topical amphotericin B. Continue systemic treatment one month after skin clears.

2) *Granulomatous Blepharoconjunctivitis:* Treat as extracutaneous disease; itraconazole 300 mg PO BID × 6 months then 200 mg PO BID long term.

[δ] Please see special note on fungal keratitis at beginning of the specific antifungal regimins

[φ] Recommend consultation with infectious disease specialist

3. Antiviral Agents

D.J. Rhee et al., *Ophthalmologic Drug Guide*, 2nd ed.,
DOI 10.1007/978-1-4419-7621-5_3,
© Springer Science+Business Media, LLC 2011

A. TOPICAL

Drug	Trade	Concentration	Usual Dose	Notes
acyclovir	Zovirax	Oint, 3%	5×/day	for HSV keratitis Not commercially available in USA but can be made by compounding pharmacies
ganciclovir	Zirgan	Gel, 0.15%	5× day until epithelium is healed, then TID× 1 week	newly approved agent for epithelial HSV for HSV conjunctivitis
idoxuridine	Herplex	Soln, 0.1%, 1% Oint, 0.5%	Q5×/day	for HSV keratitis; No longer commercially produced in USA, but can be ordered through compounding pharmacies
trifluridine	Viroptic	Soln, 1.0%	9×/day, for 7–10 days; probably as effective used	First line agent for HSV keratitis
vidarabine	Vira-A	Oint, 3.0%	5×/day 5× daily	for HSV conjunctivitis for HSV keratitis; no longer available commercially but can be made by compounding pharmacies

Note: The compounds no longer available commercially can be obtained from compounding pharmacies such as Leiter's Rx Ophthalmic Compounding Pharmacy in San Jose, CA.

B. SYSTEMIC

Note: All have significant side effects which need to be monitored; refer to insert below.

Drug	Trade	Dose	Notes
acyclovir	Zovirax	400 mg PO BID indefinitely	for prevention of recurrent HSV keratitis
		400 mg PO 3–5×/day for 7–10 days	for HSV keratitis/dermatitis
		800 mg PO 5× day for 7–10 days	for VZV ophthalmicus (if within 72 hours of rash onset)
		5 mg/kg IV Q 8 hrs × 7–10 days	for HSV in immuno-compromised patient, adjust dose in renal failure$^\kappa$
		10 mg/kg IV Q 8 hrs × 7–14 days	for primary/disseminated VZV adjust dose in renal failure$^\kappa$
		1500 mg/m^2/day IV in 3 divided doses × 7–10 days	for **Acute Retinal Necrosis**$^\tau$ should consider chronic oral suppressive dose; adjust dose in renal failure$^\kappa$
cidofovir	Vistide	5 mg/kg IV Q week for 2 weeks then 3–5 mg/kg Q 2 weeks	for CMV retinitis in HIV + patients; hydration and probenicid$^\zeta$ must be given with both intravit and IV; adjust dose in renal failure$^\kappa$; renal function with serum creatinine and urine protein must be monitored within 48 hours before each dose and dose modified granulocytopenia – monitor neutrophil counts contraindicated if serum creatinine >1.5 mg/dl, creat clearance <55 ml/min, urine protein > 100 mg/dl
famciclovir	Famvir	500 mg PO TID × 7 days	for VZV ophthalmicus (if within 72 hours of rash onset); must adjust dose in renal failure
		250–500 mg PO BID indefinitely	for prevention of recurrent HSV keratitis

(continued)

B. SYSTEMIC (*continued*)

Drug	Trade	Dose	Notes
foscarnet	Foscavir	IV induction 90 mg/kg Q 12 hrs (infuse over 1.5–2 hrs) for 2–3 weeks or 60 mg/kg (infuse over 1 hr) Q 8 hrs for 2–3 weeks IV maintenance 90–120 mg/kg (infuse over 2 hrs) QD for 5–7 days/week Intravitreal induction 1.2 mg in 0.05 ml 2–3×/week Intravitreal maintenance 1.2 mg in 0.05 ml Q week 40 mg/kg IV Q 8–12 hrs (infuse over 1 hour)	for CMV retinitis in HIV+ patients; must adjust IV dose in renal failure$^\kappa$; hydration reduces risk of nephrotoxicity; do not administer by bolus IV infusion – must use infusion pump. for HSV infection not responsive to acyclovir
ganciclovir	Cytovene	IV induction 5 mg/kg BID × 2–3 weeks IV maintenance 5 mg/kg QD × 7 days/week or 6 mg/kg QD 5 days/week Intravitreal (low dose) 200 µg in 0.1 ml (induction) 2–3×/wk for 2–3 weeks, then 200 µg in 0.1 ml Q wk (maintenance)	for CMV retinitis in HIV+ patients, must adjust dose in renal failure$^\kappa$ caution when administering ganciclovir and AZT because both drugs cause anemia and neutropenia do not administer if absolute neutrophil count <500 cells/µl or if platelet count <25,000 cells/µl

		Intravitreal (high dose) 2000 μg in 0.1 ml (induction) 2×/wk for 3 weeks, then 2000 μg in 0.1 ml Q wk (maintenance) (Ophthalmology 1998;105:1404–10) PO maintenance 1000–1500 mg TID with food	Oral ganciclovir in conjunction with a ganciclovir implant reduces the incidence of CMV retinitis (NEJM 1999;340:1063–70) (Arch. Ophthalmol. 1994;112:1531–1539)
	Vitrasert	Sustained release intraocular implant 4.5 mg (1 μg/hr) Continue therapy for 32 weeks or until progression of disease despite implant	
valacyclovir	Valtrex	1.0 Gm PO TID × 7–14 days	for VZV ophthalmicus (within 72 hours of rash onset), 3–5× more bioavailable than acyclovir, not advised in immuno-compromised patients due to thrombocytopenic purpura; must adjust dose in renal failure
		500 mg PO BID or 1 Gm PO QD indefinitely	For prevention of recurrent HSV keratitis, uveitis and retinitis
valganciclovir	Valcyte	900 mg PO BID × 3 weeks then maintenance therapy with 900 mg PO QD	Has replaced ganciclovir as the primary systemic treatment for CMV retinitis

κ For renal dosing, see Appendix 4

τ For Acute Retinal Necrosis, consider addition of systemic steroids and possibly anticoagulation (controversial)

ξ Probenicid should be given 2 Gm PO 3 hrs prior to cidofovir infusion and 1 Gm at 2 and 8 hrs post infusion

Side Effects:

Drug	Preparation	Side Effects
acyclovir	PO IV	GI disturbances, rash, headache, elevated creatinine, confusion reversible crystalline nephropathy (avoidable with adequate oral hydration), phlebitis, hallucinations, seizures, coma, encephalopathy, rash
cidofovir	Intravit IV	hypotony, iritis (causing posterior synechia and cataract), (Ophthalmology 1997;104:1827–37) – intravitreal administration no longer recommended nephrotoxicity, iritis, hypotony, neutropenia, metabolic acidosis.
famciclovir	IV PO	headache, nausea, fatigue
foscarnet	IV	renal impairment, Ca, K, Phos & Mg abnormalities, seizures, anemia, fever, nausea, diarrhea, headache, neutropenia.
ganciclovir	IV	myelosuppression, thrombocytopenia, liver function abnormalities, renal dysfunction, headaches, GI upset, psychiatric disturbances, seizure, anemia, inhibition of spermatogenesis, teratogen; do **not** give in conjunction with AZT (worsens neutropenia)
valacyclovir	PO	possible association with thrombotic thrombocytopenic purpura/hemolytic uremia syndrome in immunocompromised host with high doses, otherwise similar to acyclovir.
valganciclovir	PO	myelosuppression, diarrhea, nausea, peripheral neuropathy

4. Anti-Parasitic Agents

D.J. Rhee et al., *Ophthalmologic Drug Guide*, 2nd ed.,
DOI 10.1007/978-1-4419-7621-5_4,
© Springer Science+Business Media, LLC 2011

A. PROTOZOA

(1) Acanthamoeba

Note: Give combination of 2–3 different drops Q 1/2 hr–2 hr can consider adding itraconazole 200 mg PO QD-BID or voriconazole 200 mg po BID

Drug	Trade	Concentration	Dose	Notes
propamidine isethionate	Brolene	Soln, 0.1%	Q1/2 hr–2 hr	First line agent; not available commercially in the US; available over the counter in the UK; can be obtained from compounding pharmacies; active against trophozoites.
polymyxin B/neomycin/ gramicidin	AK-Spore, Neosporin, Ocu-spor G, Polymycin	Soln, 10,000 u/ 0.35%/0.025%	Q1/2 hr–2 hr	Second line agent; significant surface toxicity
polyhexamethylene biguanide (PHMB)	Baquacil	Soln, 0.02%	Q1/2 hr–2 hr	First line agent; not available commercially in the US; can be obtained from compounding pharmacies; active against cysts and trophozoites
chlorhexidine		Soln, 0.02%	Q1/2 hr–2 hr	First line agent; not available commercially in the US; can be obtained from compounding pharmacies; active against cysts and trophozoites
clotrimazole		Susp, 1%	Q1–2 hr	Second line agent
dibromopropamidine isethionate	Brolene	Oint, 0.15%	QHS	To be used during taper of Brolene drops; not available commercially in US
itraconazole	Sporanox	200 mg	PO BID	
voriconazole	Vfend	200 mg	PO BID	

(2) Leishmaniasis

Note: Eyelid lesion can cause conjunctivitis (*The Medical Letter*, 37:99–106, 1995)

stibogluconate sodium	Pentostam	20 Sb/kg/d IV or IM for 20–28 days
OR		
meglumine antimonate	Glucantime	20 Sb/kg/d IV or IM for 20–28 days

Note: Pediatric dosing same for both medications

(3) Microsporidia (*Encephalitozoon hellem, Nosema corneum*)

fumagillin	Fumidil-B	(Am J. of Ophthalmology 1993;115:293)
OR		
itraconazole		(Ophthalmology 1991;98:196)

Note: Infections by *E. hellem* have responded to above. No topical regimen exists for *N. corneum* – may need penetrating keratoplasty.

(4) *Pneumocystis carinii* choroiditis

trimethoprim/ sulfamethoxazole	Bactrim	20 mg/kg IV QD (of TMP component) × 21 days
OR		
pentamidine		4 mg/kg IV QD × 21 days

Note: Seen with disseminated disease. Must include systemic evaluation for other sites of disease and immunocompromised status. Pediatric dosing is the same.

(5) Toxoplasmosis retinochoroiditis (*Toxoplasma gondii*)

Drug	Trade	Dosing for Acute Infection	Maintenance
pyrimethamine	Daraprim	200 mg PO load, then 50–75 mg PO QD × 4–6 weeks	50–75 mg PO QD
PLUS sulfadiazine[ω]		1–1.5 Gm PO or IV Q 6 hrs × 4–6 weeks	500 mg–1 Gm PO Q6 hrs
PLUS folinic acid[▽]		10 mg PO 3 times per week × 4–6 weeks	10 mg PO QD
Other Alternatives clindamycin (may substitute if sulfa allergic)		300–600 mg PO QID or 900 mg IV QID × 4–6 weeks	300 mg PO QID
Note: May consider concurrent treatment with oral prednisone (1 mg/kg/day) for inflammation			
trimethoprim/sulfamethoxazole	Bactrim	10/50 mg/kg/day PO divided BID single drug therapy with TMP/SMX was as effective as combination therapy with pyrimethamine and sulfadiazine in a prospective, randomized trial (Ophthalmology 2005;112:1876–1882)	
PLUS clarithromycin		1 Gm PO BID	
PLUS azithromycin dapsone	Zithromax	1.2–1.5 Gm PO TID 100 mg PO QD	
OR			

atovaquone   Mepron   750 mg PO QID

take medicine with food to increase absorption

single drug therapy was effective in phase 1 trial; prednisone 40 mg PO QD was begun on day 3 (Ophthalmology 1999;106:148–153)

Notes: 1) May consider concurrent treatment with oral prednisone (1 mg/kg/day) for inflammation especially if optic nerve or macula involved

2) Treat for 4–6 weeks after resolution of signs/symptoms and continue folinic acid one week beyond the discontinuation of pyrimethamine therapy

(a) *Pediatric*

pyrimethamine   Daraprim   2 mg/kg/d × 3 days then 1 mg/kg/day (max 25 mg/day) × 4 weeks

PLUS

sulfadiazine[ω]   100–200 mg/kg/day × 4 weeks

PLUS

folinic acid[▽]   10 mg PO QD × 4 weeks

Note: Congenitally infected newborns should be treated with pyrimethamine and sulfadiazine every 2–3 days for one year

(b) *Pregnancy*

spiramycin   Rovamycine   3–4 grams/day × 3–4 weeks

Note: Intravitreal clindamycin 1.0 mg is another treatment option in pregnant women with ocular toxoplasmosis.

[ω]If sulfa allergic, may substitute with clindamycin

[▽]Folinic acid is used to avoid pyrimethamine-induced myelosuppression

B. HELMINTHS

(1) Filariasis (*The Medical Letter*, 1189:1–12, 2004)

(a) *Onchocerciasis (Onchocerca volvulus)*, "*river blindness*"

Drug	Trade	Dose
ivermectin	Mectizan	150 µg/kg × 1, repeated every 6–12 months until asymptomatic

Notes: 1) Consider antihistamines or corticosteroids to reduce allergic reaction caused by dead microfilaria
2) Pediatric dosing is the same

(b) *Loasis (loa loa)*

Drug	Trade	Dose	Notes
diethylcarbamazine	Hetrazan	6 mg/kg in 3 doses × 14 days	Pediatric Dose the same

Notes: 1) Heavy filaria burden may induce encephalopathy; may use ivermectin or albendazole or apheresis to reduce microfilarial counts (Infect Dis Clin North Am, 7:619, 1993).
2) Consider antihistamines or corticosteroids to reduce allergic reaction caused by dead microfilaria ("Mazzotti reaction")

(2) Tapeworm (*Taenia solium*), "Cysticercosis"

Notes:
1) Anti-helminth treatment is usually not indicated for isolated conjunctival or retinal disease, but is indicated for orbital involvement.
2) Consider obtaining CT scan to rule out neurocystercercosis, especially if anti-helminth medications are going to be used since inflammation secondary to death of organism can be fatal.
3) Isolated conjunctival involvement may be treated with surgical excision alone.
4) For posterior segment involvement, laser of worm or vitrectomy to remove organism may be preferable.
5) Anti-helminth medical regimens for orbital involvement are not standardized, but some regimens are described. Combination of albendazole or praziquantel in conjunction with prednisone (to decrease inflammation) for four weeks has been recommended (*Ophthalmology* 104; vol 10 p. 1599–1604. 1997), although single dose praziquantel has also been described (*The Medical Letter*, 1189:1–12, 2004).

albendazole	Zentel	15 mg/kg/day PO × 4 weeks	*Ophthalmol.* 104;(10) 1599–1604. 1997) Pediatric dosing same.
praziquantel	Biltricide	5–10 mg/kg once	*The Medical Letter*, 1189:1–12, 2004 Pediatric dosing same
prednisone		1.5–2.0 mg/kg/day × 4 weeks	

(3) Toxocariasis Visceral Larva Migrans (*T. canis*)

Drug	Trade	Dose	Notes
albendazole	Zentel	400 mg PO BID × 3–5 days	Pediatric dosing same
thiabendazole		25 mg/kg PO BID × 3–5 days	Pediatric dosing same

Note: Treatment with albendazole may cause an intense inflammatory reaction as the worm dies and require concurrent steroid use.

5. Anti-Glaucoma Agents

D.J. Rhee et al., *Ophthalmologic Drug Guide*, 2nd ed.,
DOI 10.1007/978-1-4419-7621-5_5,
© Springer Science+Business Media, LLC 2011

A. ALPHA AGONISTS$^{\Sigma}$ (WHITE TOP – IOPIDINE; PURPLE TOP – ALPHAGAN)

Mechanism of Action:	Activation of alpha-2 receptors in ciliary body inhibits aqueous secretion. Brimonidine also reported to increase uveoscleral outflow
Side Effects:	Local irritation, allergy, mydriasis, dry mouth, dry eye, hypotension, lethargy
Contraindications:	MAO inhibitor use

Drug	Trade	Concentration	Usual Dose	Notes
apraclonidine	Iopidine	Soln, 0.5%	TID	for short term use
		Soln, 1%	single dose	for prophylaxis of post-laser IOP spike
brimonidine	Alphagan-P	Soln, 0.1% or 0.15%	TID/BID	highly selective alpha-2 agonist may cause apnea in children
	(generic)	Soln, 0.15% or 0.2%	TID/BID	highly selective alpha-2 agonist may cause apnea in children
	Combigan	Soln, 0.2%	BID	Combigan is a combination agent with timolol – see **combination agents** listed below

$^{\Sigma}$For listing of preservatives of anti-glaucoma medications, refer to Appendix 5

B. BETA BLOCKERS$^{\Sigma}$ (0.25% – LIGHT BLUE TOP, 0.5% – YELLOW TOP)

Mechanism of action:	Beta blockade in ciliary body reduces intraocular pressure by decreasing aqueous humor production
Side Effects:	*Local:* Blurred vision, corneal anesthesia, superficial punctate keratitis *Systemic:* Bradycardia/heart block, bronchospasm, fatigue, mood change, impotence, decreases sensitivity to hypoglycemic symptoms in insulin dependent diabetics, worsening of myasthenia gravis
Contraindications:	Asthma, severe COPD, bradycardia, heart block, CHF, myasthenia gravis

Drug	Trade	Concentration	Usual Dose	Notes
betaxolol	Betoptic S	Soln, 0.25%	BID	relatively cardioselective
	Betoptic	Soln, 0.5%	BID	relatively cardioselective
carteolol	Carteolol HCl	Soln, 1%	BID	non-selective, has intrinsic sympathomimetic activity
levobetaxolol	Betaxon	Soln, 0.5%	BID	relatively cardioselective
levobunolol	AKBETA, Betagan, Levobunolol HCl	Soln, 0.25, 0.5%	QD-BID	non-selective (long half life)
metipranolol	Optipranolol	Soln, 0.3%	BID	non-selective (WHITE top)
timolol hemihydrate	Betimol	Soln, 0.25, 0.5%	BID	non-selective
timolol	Timoptic	Soln, 0.25, 0.5%	BID	non-selective
maleate	Timoptic XE	Soln, 0.25, 0.5%	QD	non-selective, gel-forming solution
	Timolol GFS			
	Istalol	Soln, 0.5%	QD	non-selective
	Cosopt	see notes	see notes	Cosopt is a combination agent with dorzolamide – see **combination agents** listed below

Σ For listing of preservatives of anti-glaucoma medications, refer to Appendix 5

C. CARBONIC ANHYDRASE INHIBITORS$^\Sigma$ (ORANGE TOP)

Mechanism of Action:	Inhibition of carbonic anhydrase decreases aqueous production in ciliary body; when given parentally, will also dehydrate the vitreous
Side Effects:	*Local (with topical therapy):* bitter taste
	Systemic (with topical therapy): diuresis, fatigue, GI upset, Stevens-Johnson syndrome, theoretical risk of aplastic anemia
	(with systemic therapy): hypokalemic/acidosis, renal stones, paresthesias, nausea, cramps, diarrhea, malaise, lethargy, depression, impotence, unpleasant taste, aplastic anemia, Stevens-Johnson syndrome
Contraindications:	sulfa allergy, hyponatremia/kalemia, recent renal stones, thiazide diuretics, digitalis use

Drug	Trade	Concentration	Usual Dose	Notes
acetazolamide	Diamox	125, 250 mg tabs	QD-QID	onset within 2 hrs, lasts 4–6 hrs
	Diamox Sequels	500 mg caps	QD-BID	lasts 12–24 hrs
		500 mg IV	one dose	immediate onset, duration 4 hrs for temporary IOP
		5–10 mg/kg/dose	PO TID-QID	control in **Infantile Glaucoma**; definitive treatment is surgical. For preparation instructions see Appendix 2. Also see subject index for further discussion.
brinzolamide	Azopt	Soln, 1%	BID-TID	TID for single therapy
dorzolamide	Trusopt	Soln, 2%	BID-TID	TID for single therapy
				BID when used in combination with beta blockers
	Cosopt	see notes	see notes	Cosopt is a combination agent with timolol maleate – see **combination agents** listed below
methazolamide	Neptazane, MZM, Glauctabs	25, 50 mg tabs	BID-QID	

$^\Sigma$For listing of preservatives of anti-glaucoma medications, refer to Appendix 5

D. HYPEROSMOLAR AGENTS[Σ]

Mechanism of Action:	Osmotically decreases intraocular fluid volume and intraocular pressure in acute situations
Side Effects:	*mannitol:* CHF, urinary retention in men, back ache, myocardial infarction, headache, mental confusion *glycerin:* vomiting, less likely to produce CHF than mannitol, otherwise similar to mannitol *isosorbide:* same as glycerin except perhaps safer in diabetes
Contraindications:	CHF, DKA (glycerin), subdural or subarachnoid hemorrhage, pre-existing severe dehydration

Drug	Trade	Concentration	Usual Dose	Notes
glycerin	Osmoglyn	50% soln	1–1.5 Gm/kg PO	Onset in 30 min, lasts 5–6 hrs
isosorbide	Ismotic	45% soln	1.5 Gm/kg PO	Onset 30–60 min, lasts 6 hrs; infuse over
mannitol	Osmitrol	5–20% soln	0.5–2 Gm/kg IV	45 minutes

[Σ]For listing of preservatives of anti-glaucoma medications, refer to Appendix 5

E. MIOTICS^Σ (GREEN TOP)

Mechanism of action:	Direct cholinergics stimulate muscarinic receptors, indirect cholinergics block acetylcholinesterase. Miotics cause pupillary muscle constriction which is believed to pull open the trabecular meshwork to increase trabecular outflow.
Side Effects:	*Direct Cholinergic Local:* brow ache, breakdown of blood/aqueous barrier, angle closure (increases pupillary block & causes the lens/iris diaphragm to move anteriorly), decreased night vision, variable myopia, retinal tear/detachment, and possibly anterior subcapsular cataracts
	Systemic: rare
	Indirect Cholinergic Local: retinal detachment, cataract, myopia, intense miosis, angle closure, increase bleeding post surgery, punctal stenosis, increase formation of posterior synechiae in chronic uveitis.
	Systemic: diarrhea, abdominal cramps, enuresis, increases effect of succinylcholine
Contraindications:	*Direct Cholinergic:* peripheral retinal pathology, central media opacity, young patient (increases myopic effect), uveitis
	Indirect Cholinergic: succinylcholine administration, predisposition to retinal tear, anterior subcapsular cataract, ocular surgery, uveitis

Drug	Trade	Concentration	Usual Dose	Notes
echothiophate iodide	Phospholine Iodide	Soln, 0.03%, 0.06%, 0.125%, 0.25%	QD-BID	indirect, avoid in phakic patients
physostigmine	Isopto Eserine Eserine	Soln, 0.25%, 0.5% Oint, 0.25%	QD-BID Unit dose	indirect, avoid in phakic patients indirect, used post-operatively
demecarium bromide	Humorsol	Soln, 0.125%, 0.25%	QD-BID	indirect
acetylcholine	Miochol-E	1:100 dilution	Inject into AC	direct, used during surgery
carbachol	Carbachol Carbastat, Miostat	Soln, 0.75, 1.5, 2.25, 3% Soln, 0.01%	QD-TID Inject into AC	direct/indirect direct/indirect, used during surgery
pilocarpine hydrochloride	Isopto Carpine, Pilocar Pilopine HS gel	Soln, 0.25%–8% Soln, 0.5, 1, 2, 3, 4, 6% Oint, 4%	QID QID QHS	direct direct direct
pilocarpine nitrate	Pilagan	Soln, 1%, 2%, 4%	QID	direct

ΣFor listing of preservatives of anti-glaucoma medications, refer to Appendix 5

F. PROSTAGLANDINS[Σ] (TEAL TOP)

Mechanism of Action:	Prostaglandin PF agonist which increases uveoscleral outflow
Side Effects:	*Local:* increase in melanin pigmentation in iris, blurred vision, eyelid redness; cystoid macular edema and anterior uveitis have been reported.
	Systemic: systemic upper respiratory infection symptoms, backache, chest pain, myalgia
Contraindications:	pregnancy; use with caution in women of child bearing potential and inform the woman of the risks to potential pregnancies; consider avoiding for uveitic glaucoma.

Drug	Trade	Bottle Size	Concentration	Usual Dose	Notes
bimatoprost	Lumigan	2.5, 5 ml	Susp, 0.01%, 0.03%	QHS	
latanoprost	Xalatan	2.5 ml	Susp, 0.005%	QHS	generic latanoprost available in the US in 2011
travoprost	Travatan-Z	2.5, 5 ml	Susp, 0.004%	QHS	Does Not require refrigeration

Note: Must be refrigerated prior to opening; good for 6 weeks once open
[Σ]For listing of preservatives of anti-glaucoma medications, refer to Appendix 5

G. SYMPATHOMIMETIC[Σ] (PURPLE TOP):

Mechanism of Action:	In ciliary body, the response is variable (beta stimulation increases aqueous production, but alpha stimulation decreases aqueous production); in trabecular meshwork, beta stimulation causes increased trabecular outflow and increased uveoscleral outflow; overall effect lowers IOP.
Side Effects:	*Local:* Cystoid macular edema in aphakia (more likely with epinephrine than dipivefrin), mydriasis, rebound hyperemia, blurred vision, adenochrome deposits, allergic blepharoconjunctivitis.
	Systemic: tachycardia/ectopy, hypertension, headache
Contraindications:	narrow angles, aphakia, pseudophakia, soft lenses, hypertension, cardiac disease

Drug	Trade	Concentration	Usual Dose	Notes
dipivefrin	Propine, Dipivefrin HCl	Soln, 0.1%	BID	prodrug of epinephrine; when initiating therapy, full effect of drug is seen 2–3 months later
epinephrine	Epifrin	Soln, 0.5, 1, 2%	BID	mixed alpha & beta agonist

[Σ]For listing of preservatives of anti-glaucoma medications, refer to Appendix 5

H. COMBINATION AGENTS[Σ]

Drug	Trade	Concentration	Usual Dose	Notes
timolol maleate/brimonidine	Combigan	Soln 0.5% / Soln 0.2%	BID	beta blocker with selective alpha-2 agonist
timolol maleate/ dorzolamide	Cosopt (generic)	Soln 0.5% / 2%	BID	beta blocker with carbonic anhydrase inhibitor
timolol maleate/latanoprost	Xalacom	Soln 0.5% / Susp 0.005%	QHS	beta blocker with prostaglandin agonist (not available in the United States)
timolol maleate/travaprost	Duotrav	Soln 0.5% / 0.004%	QD	beta blocker with prostaglandin agonist (not available in the United States)
timolol maleate/bimatoprost	Ganfort	Soln 0.4% / 0.03%	QD	beta blocker with prostaglandin agonist (not available in the United States)

[Σ]For listing of preservatives of anti-glaucoma medications, refer to Appendix 5

I. SPECIFIC REGIMENTS

(1) Infantile/Congenital Glaucoma

Notes: 1) Definitive treatment is surgical (i.e. goniotomy, trabeculotomy, trabeculectomy, tube shunt, etc.) which should be performed as soon as possible.

2) Medical treatment is done only temporarily until appropriate surgery can be performed or to clear the cornea to aid in surgical management.

3) For initial medical treatment, we use oral acetazolamide 5–10 mg/kg/dose TID-QID (for preparation instructions, see Appendix 2). This may be supplemented with timolol alone (Diagnosis and therapy of the glaucoma, sixth ed., p 605–623. C.V. Mosby Co. St. Louis) or with timolol and pilocarpine 2% (Acta Ophthalmol. Scand. 1995: 73: 261–263); in patients younger than 2 years of age, consider using 0.25% timolol rather than 0.5% to limit systemic adsorpsion Topical dorzolamide

TID is also well tolerated in patients less than 6 years of age (Arch Ophthalmol 2005;123:1177–1186). Brimonidine should be avoided in children particularly those less than 20 kg in body weight and younger than 6 years (Ophthalmology 2005;112:2143–2148); apnea has been reported (J Pediatr 2002;140:485–486, J AAPOS 2001;5:281–284, & J Pediatr 2001;138:441–443). Brimonidine is not recommended in children less than 2 years of age.

4) One report describes the relative safety of apraclondine in a series of children where 70% of the cases were less than 12 months old. However, the majority of patients were only treated for less than 20 doses i.e., very short term. (J. Glaucoma 2009;18:395–398.

5) Consultation with either an ophthalmologist specializing in either pediatrics or glaucoma is recommended.

(2) Elevated Eye Pressure During Pregnancy

Notes: 1) All medications have the potential to cause embryonic and fetal harm and should be used with extreme caution and under the supervision of a glaucoma specialist whenever possible.

2) In general, the IOP lowers during pregnancy (Chin J Physiol 1995;38:229–234 and Acta Obstet Gynecol Scand 1996;75:816–819)

3) Argon laser trabeculoplasty or selective laser trabeculoplasty can be considered first line treatments despite the lower potential for success. If possible, selective laser trabeculoplasty is favored since post-surgical anti-inflammatories should be avoided.

4) If laser trabeculoplasty fails, cyclophotocoagulation (Br. J Ophthalmol 2002;86:1318–1319) or medical management should be carefully weighed. Trabeculectomy WITHOUT anti-metabolites or post-operative anti-inflammatories can also be considered.

5) Brimonidine is classified as category B, however, stop brimonidine within one month of delievery. Other anti-glaucoma medications are generally classified category C.

6) Oral acetazolamide has been reported to be safe in a small case series for the treatment of intracranial hypertension (Am J Ophthalmol 2005;139:855–859), thus topical carbonic anhydrase inhibitors may be safe. However, acetazolamide during late pregnancy has been associated with renal tubular acidosis in the newborn and may have potential teratogenic effects if administed during the first 12 weeks of fetal development (Surv Ophthalmol 2001;45:449–454).

7) Prostaglandin analogues should be AVOIDED. Anti-metabolites should be AVOIDED.

Note: Medication safety categories from the United States Food and Drug Administration (FDA)

Category A: safety established using human studies

Category B: presumed safety based on animal studies

Category C: uncertain safety; no human studies; animal studies show adverse effect

Category D: unsafe; evidence of risk that in certain clinical circumstances may be justifiable

Category X: highly unsafe.

(3) Acute Angle Closure Glaucoma

Notes:
1) Regimen outlined below is once acute angle closure glaucoma secondary to pupillary block has been established.
2) Definitive treatment is surgical (i.e. laser iridectomy, surgical iridectomy, etc.)
3) Medical treatment is needed to facilitate surgical management.
4) Unless contraindicated, we use topical agents (beta blockers, alpha agonists, and carbonic anhydrase inhibitors), systemic carbonic anhydrase inhibitors (do not use sustained release Diamox Sequels), hyperosmolar agents, and topical steroids
   a) topical Agents
      one drop of a beta blocker – timolol maleate or levobunolol 0.5%
      one drop of an alpha agonist – apraclonidine 1.0% or brimonidine 0.2%
      one drop of dorzolamide 2% or brinzolamide 1%
      one drop of prednisolone acetate 1% Q 15–30 minutes for four doses then hourly
   b) systemic Agents
      one dose of acetazolamide 250–500 mg orally
5) Recheck the IOP and visual acuity in one hour. If the IOP does not lower and the vision does not improve, we repeat the topical medications and give mannitol 1–2 g/kg IV over 45 minutes (a 500 ml bag of mannitol 20% contains 100 g of mannitol).
6) Once the IOP is lowered, laser iridectomy can be attempted. If IOP does not lower or view is too poor for performing a laser iridectomy, then a surgical iridectomy or guarded filtration procedure may be required.

6. Neuro-Ophthalmology

D.J. Rhee et al., *Ophthalmologic Drug Guide*, 2nd ed.,
DOI 10.1007/978-1-4419-7621-5_6,
© Springer Science+Business Media, LLC 2011

A. AGENTS USED IN NEURO-OPHTHALMOLOGY

Drug	Trade	Preparation	Usual Dose	Notes
botulinum toxin	Botox	Injection	Varies depending on the entity being treated	Used in treatment of blepharospasm, strabismus, and hemifacial spasm
cocaine	N/A	Soln, 10%	1 drop, repeat in 1 minute	Used in diagnosis of Horner's syndrome[†]
edrophonium chloride	Tensilon	IV Soln, 10 mg/ml	2–3 mg IV (0.2–0.3 cc)*	Used in diagnosis of Myasthenia Gravis; if unresponsive and no side effects seen after 1 min., may give 0.4 cc Q 30 sec × 2
hydroxyamphetamine	Paredrine	Soln, 1%	1 drop, repeat in 1 minute	Used in diagnosis of Horner's syndrome.* No longer available in US
methylprednisolone	Solu-Medrol	IV Soln	250 mg IV Q 6 hrs	Treatment of optic neuritis and giant cell arteritis (see below for further discussion)
			Special (See Below)	Traumatic optic neuropathy "Traumatic optic neuropathy"
pilocarpine	N/A	Soln, 0.125%	1 drop	Lower strength used in diagnosis and treatment of Adie's pupil[†]

*Potential for causing cholinergic crisis, treatment of which includes IV atropine

B. SPECIFIC REGIMENS

(1) Giant Cell Arteritis

Notes: 1) Opinions on treatment varies between rheumatologists and among neuro-ophthalmologists. Some feel oral prednisone10 mg BID is sufficient (J. Rheumatol. 1990;17:1340–1345). Others have written that if no visual symptoms have occurred, oral prednisone 60–80 mg QD (Ann Intern. Med. 1978;188:162–167, Surv Ophthalmol. 1976;20:547–260, and Am. Heart J. 1980;100:99–107 as discussed in Arch. Fam. Med. 1994;3:623–627) is adequate.

2) Most patients have visual symptoms and we recommend high dose intravenous methylprednisolone (Arch. Fam. Med. 1994;3:623–627).

Drug	Trade	Preparation	Dosage
methylprednisolone	Solu-Medrol	IV Soln	250 mg IV Q 6 hrs x 3 days day 4: begin taper with oral prednisone

(2) Optic Neuritis[γ]

Notes: 1) Intravenous steroids may speed the recovery of visual acuity.
2) Oral steroids do not hasten recovery time of visual acuity and may worsen the relapse rate.

Drug	Trade	Preparation	Dosage
methylprednisolone	Solu-Medrol	IV Soln	250 mg IV Q 6 hrs × 3 days (N. Eng. J. Med. 329: 1764–1769, day 4: begin taper with oral prednisone Dec. 9, 1993) 1 mg/kg/day for 11 days then, 4 day taper of oral prednisone (20 mg, 10 mg, 0 mg, then 10 mg)

(3) Traumatic Optic Neuropathy[γ]

Notes: 1) This is an experimental alternative protocol to decompressive surgery; definitive treatment has not been established
(Seminars in Ophthalmology, Vol. 9, No. 3 (Sept), 1994: pp 200–211)

Drug	Trade	Dose	Notes
methylprednisolone	Solu-Medrol	IV Soln	30 mg/kg IV load (2 Gm for healthy adult), then **either** 4.0 mg/kg/hr continuous IV infusion × 24 hrs **or** additional 15 mg/kg 2 hrs later and 15 mg/kg (1 Gm in healthy adults) Q6 hrs × 72 hour

(4) Pseudotumor cerebri

Notes: 1) Treatment is not indicated in all cases. Consider treatment if there is evidence of visual acuity or visual field decline or severe headaches.

2) Weight loss is a very important component of treatment if the patient is overweight.

Drug	Trade	Dose	Notes
acetazolamide	Diamox	250 mg PO QID	Slowly build up to 500 mg PO QID if tolerated. Acetazolamide is a sulfa containing medication

[γ]Consultation with neuro-ophthalmologist is recommended for duration of taper

7. Anti-Inflammatory Agents

D.J. Rhee et al., *Ophthalmologic Drug Guide*, 2nd ed.,
DOI 10.1007/978-1-4419-7621-5_7,
© Springer Science+Business Media, LLC 2011

A. STEROIDAL

Notes: 1) Suspensions are more lipophilic and penetrate the cornea more easily that solutions
2) Relative anti-inflammatory potency as follows:

Intravenous or intravitreal		Topical	
cortisone	0.8	low potency:	cortisone
cortisol (endogenous)	1		hydrocortisone
hydrocortisone (synthetic)	1	mild potency:	fluorometholone
prednisone	4		medrysone
prednisolone	4	moderate potency:	fluorometholone acetate
methylprednisolone	5		dexamethasone phosphate
triamcinolone	5		rimexolone
betamethasone	25	high potency:	loteprednol etabonate
dexamethasone	25	higher potency:	prednisolone phosphate
fluorometholone	40–50		dexamethasone acetate
		highest potency	prednisolone acetate
			difluprednate

(1) Topical

Drug	Trade	Preparation	Usual Dosage
			used primarily for dermatologic/rheumatologic conditions
cortisone	Cortone		variable
dexamethasone acetate	AK-Dex, Decadron	Susp, 0.1%	variable
	AK-Dex, Decadron	Oint, 0.05%	variable
dexamethasone phosphate	Decadron, AK-Dex	Soln, 0.1%	
difluprednate	Durezol	Emulsion, 0.05%	QID but dose varies (QID dosing equivalent to prednisolone 8 times per day for uveitis)*
fluorometholone	Fluro-op, FML	Susp, 0.1%	QOD-QID
	FML Forte	Susp, 0.25%	QOD-QID
	FML S.O.P.	Oint, 0.1%	QD-QID
fluorometholone acetate	Eflone, Flarex	Susp, 0.1%	QOD-QID
hydrocortisone	exists only in combination with antibiotic		
loteprednol etabonate	Alrex	Susp, 0.2%	QD-QID
	Lotemax	Susp, 0.5%	variable
medrysone	HMS	Susp, 1%	QD-Q4 hrs
prednisolone acetate	Pred Mild	Susp, 0.12%	variable
	Econopred	Susp, 0.125%	variable
	Pred Forte, Econopred Plus	Susp, 1%	variable
prednisolone phosphate	AKPred, Inflammase Mild, Pred-Phosphate	Soln, 0.125%	variable
	AKPred, Inflammase Forte, Pred-Phosphate	Soln, 1%	variable
rimexolone	Vexol	Susp, 1%	variable

* Jamal KN and Callanan DG. Clinical Ophthalmology 2009;3:381–390

(2) Subtenons/Intravitreal/Systemic

Drug	Trade	Preparation	Usual Dosage	Notes
triamcinolone	Kenalog Triescence Trivaris	40 mg/ml 40 mg/ml 80 mg/ml	0.5–1.0 ml for SubTenon's 0.1 ml total vol for intravitreal to a total dose typically between 4–25 mg	subtenons or intravitreal for uveitis and CME; lasts weeks to months; Triescence and Trivaris are preservative-free formulations. Also used for vitreous visualization during vitrectomy
betamethasone	Celestone	6 mg/ml	0.5–1.0 ml	subtenons post-cataract surgery, corneal transplant, uveitis, and CME; last few days to one week
dexamethasone acetate	N/A		0.4 mg in 0.1 ml	intravitreal injection for endophthalmitis
dexamethasone intravitreal implant	Ozurdex	Intravitreal implant	0.7 mg	Approved for treatment of macular edema secondary to branch or central retinal vein occlusion and uveitis. Injected intravitreally as outpatient procedure. Lasts 2–4 months.
fluocinolone acetonide intravitreal implant	Retisert	Intravitreal implant	0.59 mg	Approved for treatment of chronic noninfectious uveitis. Inserted at pars plana in operating room. Lasts 3 years.
methylprednisolone	Depo-Medrol, Solu-Medrol	IV Soln		See subject index for further discussion of giant cell arteritis, optic neuritis, and traumatic optic neuropathy
prednisone		1,2.5,5,10,20,50 mg tabs	variable	

B. COMBINATION STEROID WITH ANTIBIOTIC

Drug	Trade	Preparation	Usual Dosage	Notes
dexamethasone acetate/neomycin/ polymyxin B	Maxitrol, Neopolydex, Ocu-trol, W-DNP	Susp, 0.1%	QD-QID	BC antibiotics with high potency steroid
dexamethasone (as salt)/ tobramycin	Tobradex	Oint, 0.1%	QD-QID	BC antibiotic with high potency steroid
dexamethasone acetate/tobramycin	Tobradex	Susp, 0.1%	QD-QID	BC antibiotic with high potency steroid
dexamethasone (as salt)/neomycin	Dexacidin	Oint, 0.1%	QD-QID	BC antibiotic with high potency steroid
dexamethasone phosphate/ neomycin	Dexacidin, Neodecadron, Neodexasone Neodecadron	Soln, 0.1% Oint, 0.5%	QD-Q 1 hr QD-QID	BC antibiotic with moderate potency steroid
fluorometholone/sulfacetamide	FML-S	Susp. 0.1%/10%	QD-QID	BS antibiotic with mild potency steroid
hydocortisone/neomycin/ polymyxin B/bacitracin	Cortimycin, Cortisporin	Susp, 1%	QD-QID	BC antibiotics with low potency steroid
hydrocortisone/neomycin/ polymyxin B	Cortimycin, Cortisporin AK-Spore HC	Oint Susp, 1%	QD-QID QD-QID	BC antibiotics with low potency steroid
hydrocortisone/neomycin/ polymyxin B/gramicidin	AK-Spore HC	Oint	QD-QID	BC antibiotics with low potency steroid

(continued)

B. COMBINATION STEROID WITH ANTIBIOTIC *(continued)*

Drug	Trade	Preparation	Usual Dosage	Notes
hydrocortisone/oxytetracycline/ polymyxin **B**	Terra-Cortril	Susp, 1.5%/ 0.5%/ 10,000 u	TID	BC antibiotics with low potency steroid
loteprednol etabonate/tobramycin	Zylet	Susp, 0.5%/0.3%	QD-QID	BC with moderate potency steroid
prednisolone acetate/gentamicin	Pred-G	Susp, 0.1%/0.3%	QD-QID	BC antibiotic with high potency steroid
	Pred-G S.O.P.	Oint, 0.6%/0.3%	QD-QID	
prednisolone acetate/neomycin/ polymyxin **B**	Poly-Pred	Susp, 0.5%	QD-QID	BC antibiotics with high potency steroid
prednisolone acetate/sulfacetamide	AK-Cide	Susp, 0.5%/10%	QD-QID	BS antibiotic with high potency steroid
prednisolone acetate/sulfacetamide	Blephamide	Susp, 0.2%/10%	QD-QID	BS antibiotic with high potency steroid
	Blephamide	Oint, 0.2%/10%	QD-QID	
prednisolone acetate/sulfacetamide	Cetapred	Susp, 0.25%/10%	QD-QID	BS antibiotic with high potency steroid
prednisolone acetate/sulfacetamide	Metimyd, Sulfamide	Susp, 0.5%/10%	QD-QID	BS antibiotic with high potency steroid
	Metimyd, Sulfamid Oint. Sulster, Vasocidin	Oint, 0.5%/10% Soln, 0.25%/10%	QD-QID QD-QID	
prednisolone phosphate/ sulfacetamide	Vasocidin	Oint, 0.5%/10%	QD-QID	BS antibiotic with moderate potency steroid

BC = bacteriocidal
BS = bacteriostatic

C. NONSTEROIDAL

Note: *Relative contraindication* – triad asthma (asthma in combination with aspirin sensitivity and nasal polyposis)

Drug	Trade	Preparation	Usual Dosage	Notes
bromfenac	Xibrom Bromday	Soln, 0.09% Soln, 0.09%	BID QD	FDA approved for pain and inflammation after cataract surgery approved for 16 day once daily dosing after cataract surgery beginning 1 day preoperatively, used on the day of surgery, and for 14 more days
diclofenac	Voltaren	Soln, 0.1%	QID	indicated for post-cataract surgery inflammation and treatment of photophobia after incision refractive surgery
flurbiprofen	Ocufen	Soln, 0.03%	2 drops @ 3,2,1 hrs before surgery	indicated for intraoperative miosis inhibition
ketorolac	Acular Acular LS	Soln, 0.5% Soln, 0.4%	QID QID	indicated for ocular itching and pain and treatment of post-cataract surgery inflammation may decrease pain after noninfected, non-contact lens-related, traumatic corneal abrasions (Ophthalmology 1997;104:1353–59)
	Acular PF	Soln, 0.5%	QID	indicated for ocular itching and post-operative pain and photophobia radial keratotomy: preservative free in unit dose vial
	Acuvail	Soln, 0.45%	BID	indicated for pain and inflammation following cataract surgery: preservative free in unit dose vial
nepafenac suprofen	Nevanac Profenal	Susp, 0.1% Soln, 1%	TID 1 drop Q 30 min starting 2 hrs before surgery	FDA approved for pain and inflammation after cataract surgery indicated for intraoperative miosis inhibition

D. MISCELLANEOUS

Drug	Trade	Preparation	Usual Dose	Notes
cyclosporine	Sandimmune, Neoral	Tablets, 25, 50, 100 mg Oral sol'n 100 mg/ml	2.5–5.0 mg/kg/ day	Used for severe uveitis in children and adolescents (Ophthalmology 1998;105:2028-34) May have significant side effects, including nephrotoxicity, hypertension, anemia, and gingival hyperplasia. Serum creatinine, hemoglobin, and blood pressure must be monitored. Drug levels may need to be monitored depending on dose given
		Soln, 2% (in oil)	QID	for **ligneous conjunctivitis** and other inflamm. conditions
			QID × 3 months	for steroid-dependent **Atopic Keratoconjunctivitis** (Ophthalmology 2004;111:476-82)
		Soln, 1% (in tears)	QD-QID	for prevention of graft rejection for inflammatory peripheral ulcerative keratitis
	Restasis	Oil emulsion 0.05%	BID	FDA approved for the treatment of dry eyes

8. Mydriatics, Cycloplegics, and Reversal Agents

D.J. Rhee et al., *Ophthalmologic Drug Guide*, 2nd ed.,
DOI 10.1007/978-1-4419-7621-5_8,
© Springer Science+Business Media, LLC 2011

Drug	Trade	Concentration	Usual Dose/Indication	Notes
atropine	Atropisol, Isopto Atropine, Ocu-tropine Ocu-tropine	Soln, 0.5,1,2,3% Oint, 1%	BID-TID (hyphema/inflammation) BID-3x/week (inflamm./pediatric refraction)	Anti-cholinergic agent Duration 7–14 days Useful in infants/children
cyclopentolate	AK-Pentolate, Cyclogel Ocu-pentolate, Pentolair	Soln, 0.5, 1, 2% Soln, 1%	TID-QID (inflammation)	Anti-cholinergic agent[#] Increased risk of CNS toxicity (psychotic rxn) in children Duration 1–2 days
dapiprazole	Rev-Eyes	Soln, 0.5%	1 drop (reverse dilation)	Alpha blocker, reverses mydriasis from phenylephrine & to lesser extent tropicamide
homatropine	Isopto Homatropine	Soln, 2, 5%	BID-TID (inflammation)	Anti-cholinergic agent[#] Duration 3 days; better for children
phenylephrine	AK-Dilate, Mydfrin, Neo-Synephrine, Ocu-phrin AK-Nefrin, Ocu-phrin	Soln, 2.5, 10% Soln, 0.12%	1 drop (mydriasis)	Adrenergic agent Duration 3–5 hours

scopolamine	Isopto Hyoscine	Soln, 0.25%	BID-TID (inflammation)	Anti-cholinergic agent[#] Duration 3–7 days; better for children
tropicamide	Mydriacyl, Ocu-tropic, Topicacyl	Soln, 0.5, 1%	1 drop (cycloplegia)	Anti-cholinergic agent[#] Duration 4–6 hours
tropicamide/ hydroxyamphetamine hydrobromide	Paremyd	Soln, 1%/0.25%	1 drop (mydriasis)	Anti-cholinergic agent[#] with adrenergic agent
scopolamine/ phenylephrine	Murocoll 2	Soln, 0.3/10%	1 drop (mydriasis)	Anti-cholinergic agent[#] with adrenergic agent

[#]Note: Anti-cholineric agents are cycloplegics

Note: Duration is in the non-inflammed eye. The duration is shorter in the inflammed eye

9. Lubricants and Viscoelastics

D.J. Rhee et al., *Ophthalmologic Drug Guide*, 2nd ed.,
DOI 10.1007/978-1-4419-7621-5_9,
© Springer Science+Business Media, LLC 2011

A. ARTIFICIAL TEARS, VISCOELASTICS, AND LUBRICATING OINTMENTS

Notes: 1) Viscosity of water is 0.7 centistokes*
2) centistokes (cs) X density = centipoits (cp)
3) centipoits • seconds = cps
4) Boric acid is a balanced salt solution used to equalize osmolarity

Preservatives Legend:

N = None	1 = Purite	2 = EDTA	3 = Benzalkonium chloride	4 = Chlorobutanol
5 = Polyquad	6 = Sorbic acid	7 = Sodium perborate	8 = Methyl propylparbens	9 = Polyhexamethylene biguanide
10 = polixetonium	N/A = Not available	11 = chlorite		

Low Viscosity

Low viscosity lubricants are useful in mildly symptomatic **dry eyes**; they have a low tendency to blur vision but typically do not last as very long.

Trade Name	Viscosity	Osmolarity	Preservative
Preservative Free			
Bion Tears	5–15 cps*** / 4.5 cs*	270–330	N
Dry Therapy	0.7 cs*	N/A	N
Hypotears PF	<5 cps⁺⁺ / 1.2 cs* / 2.8 cp**	220	N
Oasis Tears	30 cp	275	N
Preservative Free Advanced Eye Relief	< 5 cps ©	270–330	N
Refresh, Optive Sensitive	5 cp** / 2.8 cs*	250–305	N
Refresh Plus	3 cp** / 2.0 cs*	270–340	N
Systane (preservative free)	7–15 cps	270–330	N

	Viscosity	Osmolarity	N
Systane Ultra Unit Dose	9–15 cps	265–290	N
Tears Naturale Free	5–15 cp*** / 4.3 cs*	270–330	N
Preserved			
AKWA Tears	3.5 cp	250–310	2, 3
Blink Tears	11 cp	175	11
Computer Eye Drops	< 5 cps©	270–330	3
FreshKote	22.5 cps	288–291	10
GenTeal	7 cps++ / 3.6 cs*	220	7
Hypotears	< 5 cps++ / 1.2 cs* / 2.8 cp**	220	2, 3
Isopto Plain	15–30 cps***	270–330	3
Isopto Tears	15–30 cps***	270–330	3
Liquifilm Tears	4 cp**	220–270	4
Advanced Eye Relief	< 5 cps©	270–330	3
Murine	2.3 cp†	260	2, 3
Optive	20 cps	330	1
Puralube Tears	5 cp††	N/A	2, 3
Refresh Tears	3.0 cp**	280	1
Soothe	2.0–2.2 cps^	240–289	9
Systane	7–15 cps©©	270–330	5
Systane Ultra	8–15 cps	270–300	5
Tearisol	10–30 cp++	220	2, 3
Tears Naturale	5–15 cp*** / 3.7 cs* / 7.0 cp**	270–330	3
Tears Naturale II	6–12 cp*** / 4.0 cs*	270–330	5
Tears Plus	4 cp** / 2.8 cs*	260–310	4
Tears Renewed	2–10 cps©©	265–325	3

Tears Naturale like no longer available, just Tears Natural Tears II and Tear Naturale Forte

High Viscosity

High viscosity lubricants are useful in severely symptomatic **dry eyes**; they have a tendency to blur vision but last longer than low viscosity products. If symptoms are not controlled by artifical tears, consider temporary or permanent punctal occlusion therapy; tarsorraphy may be considered for severe cases of exposure keratopathy.

Trade Name	Viscosity	Osmolarity	Preservative
Preservative Free			
Aquasite PF	250–750 cps^{++} / 800 cp**	235	N
Celluvisc	170 cs* / 200–300 cp**	270–350	N
Oasis Tears Plus	>100 cp	300	N
Ocucoat PF	46 cs*	285 ± 32	N
Refresh Endura	150 cps	220–300	N
Preserved			
Aquasite	250–750 cps^{++} / 800 cp**	235	2
Blink Gel Tears	50 cp	175	11
Ocucoat	46 cs*	285 ± 32	3
Ultra Tears	100–300 cps***	270–330	3

Unknown Viscosity

Trade Name	Viscosity	Osmolarity	Preservative
Comfort Tears	N/A	N/A	2, 3
Dry Eyes Lubricant Eye Drops	N/A	N/A	3
Dwelle	N/A	N/A	10
Murocel	N/A	N/A	8
Ocu-Tears PF	N/A		N
Theratears	N/A	170	N
Visine Tears	N/A	270–320	3
Visine Pure Tears Portables	N/A		N

Insert

Drug	Trade Name	Preparation	Usual Dose	Notes
hydroxypropyl cellulose	Lacrisert	Insert, 5 mg	QD-BID	for moderate to severe **dry eye** syndrome

Gels & Ointments

Ointments

Trade Name	Notes
	Note: Some individuals may be allergic to lanolin
AKWA Tears Ointment	Lanolin containing
Dry Eyes	not available
Dry Eyes Lubricant Ointment	Lanolin containing
Duolube	Lanolin free
Duratears Naturale	Lanolin containing
Hypotears	Lanolin free
Lacri-Gel	Lanolin containing
Lacri-Lube S.O.P	Lanolin containing
Lubefree Petrolatum, Mineral Oil Lubricant	Lanolin free
LubriTears Lubricant Eye Ointment	Lanolin containing
Moisture Eyes PM	Lanolin free
Ocu-Lube	Lanolin containing
Puralube	Lanolin free
Refresh P.M.	Lanolin containing
Systane Nightime Ointment	Lanolin containing
Tears Renewed Ointment	Lanolin free

Gels

Trade Name	Notes
GenTeal Lubricant Eye Gel$^{\Omega}$	contains carbopol 980, claimed to transform from gel to liquid upon contact with the eye
Night & Day Tears Again Sterile Lubricant Gel	contains povidone 0.1% therefore is not recommended for people with iodine allergies; preserved with benzalkonium chloride; not recommended for contact lens wearing patients

Viscoelastics

SH = sodium hyaluronate
HMC = hydroxymethylcellulose
CS = chondroitin sulfate

adapative: molecules fracture when exposed to high shear rates

Trade Name	Component	Viscosity	Molecular Weight	Cohesive versus Dispersive
Amvisc	1.2% SH	40,000 cSt (62,000 cp^{+})	2,000,000 daltons	cohesive
Amvisc Plus	1.6% SH	55,000 cSt (82,000 cp^{+})	1,500,000 daltons	cohesive
BioLon	1.0% SH	215,000 cps$^{\Delta}$	3,000,000 daltons	cohesive
Cellugel	2.0% HMC	20,000–40,000 cps	300,000 daltons	dispersive
CoEase	1.2% SH	40,000 cps	1,000,000 daltons	cohesive
DuoVisc				
EyeVisc	2.0% HMC	4,000 cps	Unknown	dispersive
EyeVisc Plus	2.0% HMC	40,000 cps	Unknown	dispersive
EyeVisc SH	1.4% SH	50,000 cps	Unknown	cohesive
Healon	1.0% SH	200,000 cp^{+}	4,000,000 daltons	cohesive

HealonGV	1.4% SH	2,000,000 cp+	5,000,000 daltons	cohesive
Healon 5	2.3% SH	7,000,000 cp	4,000,000 daltons	cohesive possibly adaptive
LensVisc MC	2.0% HMC	4,000 mPas	86,000 daltons	dispersive
LensVisc HA	2.0% SH	>10,000 mPas	2,300,000 daltons	cohesive
Occu-Lon	1.5% SH	50,000 cps	2,000,000 daltons	dispersive
Ocucoat	2.0% HMC	4,000 cp+	80,000 daltons	cohesive
Provisc	1.0% SH	135,000 cp+	1,900,000 daltons	cohesive
STAARVisc II	1.2% SH	40,000 cps		cohesive
UniVisc	1.0% SH	Unknown	3,000,000 daltons	cohesive
Viscoat	3.0% SH and 4% CS in a 3:1 ratio	50,000 cp+	22,500 daltons for chondroitin sulfate and 500,000 daltons sodium hyaluronate	dispersive
Vitrax	3.0 % SH	35,000 cp+	500,000 daltons	dispersive

+ 37 C shear rate 0/sec (provided by Pharmacia advertisement)
+ + Measured on Brookfield Digital Cone and Plate Viscometer (provided by CIBA file data)
A provided by Akorn file data
* 37 C measured on Cannon-Fenske Viscometer (provided by Stortz advertisement)
** 25 C shear rate 2.6/sec (provided by Allergan file data)
*** 25 C measured on Brookfield Digital Cone and Plate Viscometer (provided by Alcon file data)
† 25 C measured on Brookfield Digital Cone and Plate Viscometer (provided by Ross file data)
†† 25 C measured on Brookfield Digital Cone and Plate Viscometer (provided by Fougera file data)
Y Provided by Allergan file data
§ Shear rate 2/sec (provided by Mentor file data)
§§ Provided by Shah & Shah IOL Ltd.
© Provided by Bausch & Lomb file data
©© Provided by Akorn file data
A Provided by Alimera Sciences, Inc.

B. IRRIGATING SOLUTIONS

Preservatives Legend:

1 = Thimerosal	2 = Benzalkonium chloride	3 = Phenylmercuric acetate

Trade Name	Preservatives
AK-Rinse	2
Blinx	3
Collyrium	1
Dacriose	2
Eye Stream	2
Iri-Sol	2
Irrigate	2
Lavoptik Eye Wash	2
M/Rinse	1

10. Miscellaneous

D.J. Rhee et al., *Ophthalmologic Drug Guide*, 2nd ed.,
DOI 10.1007/978-1-4419-7621-5_10,
© Springer Science+Business Media, LLC 2011

A. AGENTS FOR RELIEF OF SEASONAL ALLERGIC CONJUNCTIVITIS/OCULAR DISCOMFORT

Drug	Trade	Preparation	Usual Dose	Notes
azelastine	Optivar	Soln, 0.05%	BID	H1-Antagonist with mast cell stabilization
bepotastine besilate	Bepreve	Soln, 1.5%	BID	H1-Antagonist, mast cell stabilizer also inhibits other cytokines
cromolyn sodium	Crolom, Opticrom	Soln, 4%	QID–Q 4 hr	Mast cell stabilizer – may take weeks for effect
emedastine difumarate	Emadine	Soln, 0.05%	QD–QID	H1-Antagonist
epinastine	Elestat	Soln, 0.05%	BID	H1, H2 Antagonist, mast cell inhibitor
ketotifen fumarate	Zaditor	Soln, 0.025%	BID–TID	H1-Antagonist, mast cell stabilizer, eosinphil inhibitor. Now over the counter
ketorolac	Acular	Soln, 0.5%	QID	Nonsteroidal anti-inflammatory agent
	Acular PF	Soln, 0.5%	QID	presevative free in unit dose vial
levocabastine	Livostin	Soln, 0.05%	BID–QID	H1-Antagonist (preservative may damage contact lenses)
loteprednol etabonate	Alrex	Soln, 0.2%	QD–QID	Corticosteroid – must monitor for steroid complications, but is considered a "soft steroid" with less IOP and cataract effects
	Lotemax	Soln, 0.5%	QD–QID	Same compound as Alrex at an increased concentration; Corticosteroid – must monitor for steroid complications, but is considered a "soft steroid" with less IOP and cataract effects
lodoxamide	Alomide	Soln, 0.1%	QID × 2–3 weeks	Mast cell inhibitor, possibly faster onset than cromolyn; still takes a few weeks for full effect
nedocromil	Alocril	Soln, 2%	BID	Mast cell stabilizer
olopatadine	Patanol	Soln, 0.1%	BID	H1-Antagonist with mast cell stabilization
	Pataday	Soln, 0.2%	QD	H1-Antagonist with mast cell stabilization
pemirolast	Alamast	Soln, 0.1%	QID	Mast cell stabilizer

B. OCULAR DECONGESTANTS

Drug	Trade	Preparation	Usual Dose	Notes
naphazoline	All Clear, Allergy Drops, Digest 2, Naphcon	Soln, 0.012%	QID PRN	alpha agonist
	All Clear AR, Comfort Eye Drops	Soln, 0.03%	QID PRN	
	AK-Con, Napha-Forte, Naphcon Forte, Nafazair, Vasocon,	Soln, 0.1%	QID PRN	
	Opcon Max. Strength, Allergy Drops			
		Soln, 0.3%	QID PRN	
naphazoline/glycerin	Clear Eyes	Soln, 0.012%/0.2%	QID PRN	alpha agonist/artificial tear
naphazoline/polyvinyl alcohol	Albalon	Soln, 0.1%/1.4%	QID PRN	alpha agonist/art. tear
	Vasoclear	Soln, 0.02%/2.5%		
naphazoline/polyvinyl alcohol/zinc sulfate	Vasoclear A	Soln, 0.02%/2.5%	QID PRN	alpha agonist/art. tear/astringent⊕
naphazoline/glycerin/zinc sulfate	Clear Eyes ACR	Soln, 0.012%/0.2%/0.25%	QID PRN	alpha agonist/art. tear/astringent⊕
naphazoline/pheiramine	Naphcon-A, Napha-A, OcuHist, Visine-A	Soln, 0.025%/0.3%	QID PRN	alpha agonist/antihistamine
naphazoline/antazoline	Vasocon-A	Soln, 0.05%/0.5%	QID PRN	alpha agonist/antihistamine
oxymetazoline	Ocuclear, Visine LR	Soln, 0.025%	QID PRN	alpha agonist
phenylephrine	AK-Nefrin, Ocu-phrin	Soln, 0.12%	QID PRN	alpha agonist

(continued)

B. OCULAR DECONGESTANTS *(continued)*

Drug	Trade	Preparation	Usual Dose	Notes
phenylephrine/ polyvinyl alcohol	Prefrin Liquifilm Vasoconstrictor & Lubricant Eye Drops	Soln, 0.12%/1.4%	QID PRN	alpha agonist/art. tear
phenylephrine/zinc sulfate	Zinefrin	Soln, 0.12%/0.25%	QID PRN	alpha agonist/ astringent⊕
tetrahydrozoline	Eye Drops Regular, Eyesine, Eye-Zine, Murine Plus, Visine Original	Soln, 0.05%	QID PRN	alpha agonist
tetrahydrozoline/zinc sulfate	Eye Drops AC, Visine AC	Soln, 0.05%/0.25%	QID PRN	alpha agonist/ astringent⊕
tetrahydrozoline/ polyethylene glycol	Visine Advanced Relief	Soln, 0.05%	QID PRN	alpha agonist/art. tear

⊕ Astringents help clear mucous by precipitating proteins

C. TOPICAL HYPEROSMOLAR AGENTS

Drug	Trade	Preparation	Usual Dose	Notes
glycerin	Ophthalgen		1 drop prior to exam	diagnostic agent used to clear edematous cornea
sodium chloride	Muro-128	Soln, 2, 5%	QD-Q3 hrs	therapeutic agent to dehydrate the cornea
	AK-NaCl, NACL 5%	Soln, 5%	QD-Q3 hrs	
	AK-NaCl, Muro-128, NACL	Oint, 5%	QD-Q3 hrs	
glucose	Glucose 40 Ophthalmic	Oint, 40%		therapeutic agent

D. VITAMINS

Drug	Trade	Preparation	Dose	Notes
see notes	MaxiVision	Liquid	1 table spoon	multivitamin, multimineral, multinutrient, colloidal minerals
see notes	MaxiVision Whole Body Formula	Capsules	1 tab PO QD	multivitamin, multimineral, multinutrient, plant derived chelated minerals, antioxidants
see notes	MaxiVision Ocular Formula	Capsules	1 tab PO QD	multivitamin, multimineral, multinutrient, antioxidants
see notes	Ocuvite	Tablets	1 tab PO QD	zinc & anti-oxidant vitamin supplement
see notes	Ocuvite Extra	Tablets	1 tab PO QD	zinc & anti-oxidant vitamin supplement with vit B, all in higher conc. than Ocuvite
see notes	Tears Again	Soln	1 spray to lids PRN	lubricant with vitamins A and E
see notes	Viva-Drops	Soln	1 drop PRN	lubricant with anti-oxidants

E. ANESTHETIC AGENTS

(1) Topical Anesthetics$^{\psi}$

Drug	Trade	Preparation	Dose	Notes
benoxinate	Fluress, Fluorox	Soln, 0.4% with 0.25% fluorescein sodium	1 drop	Duration 15–30 min, Ester linkage, preserved with chlorobutanol
cocaine hydrochloride	N/A	Soln, 1%–4%	1 drop	Duration 20–45 min, pupillary dilation, potentiates epinephrine
paracaine	OCuSOFT	Soln, 0.5%	1 drop	
proparacaine	AK-Taine, Alcaine, Ocu-Caine, Ophthaine, Ophthetic	Soln, 0.5%	1 drop	Duration 15–30 min. Ester linkage, Ophthetic preserved with benzalkonium chloride
	Fluorocaine	Soln, 0.5% with 0.25% fluorescein sodium	1 drop	
tetracaine	AK-T-Caine, Pontocaine	Soln, 0.5%	1 drop	Duration 9–24 min. Ester linkage

Notes: 1) Topical anesthetics should **only** be used to allow the clinician to perform ocular procedures. They are **not** indicated for use by the patient and should **never** be prescribed.

2) Allergies to topical anesthetic drops may be a reaction to the medication itself, class of linkage (e.g. amide versus ester), or simply the preservative.

(2) Local Anesthetics$^\psi$ (To convert percent solutions to mg/ml, multiply by 10; e.g. 1% = 10 mg/ml)

Drug	Trade	Preparation	Maximum Adult Dose	Duration of Action	Pain on Injection[x]	Linkage[∞]
bupivacaine	Marcaine, Sensorcaine	Soln, 0.25–0.75%	23 ml of 0.75% soln	3 to 12 hrs	5	Amide
chloroprocaine	Nesacaine	Soln, 1–3%	40 ml of 2% soln	60 min	N/A	Ester
etidocaine	Duranest	Soln, 1%	40 ml of 1% soln	5–10 hrs	N/A	Amide
hexylcaine		Soln, 1–2%		60 min	N/A	Ester
lidocaine	Xylocaine					Amide
Without epinephrine		Soln, 1–2%	15 ml of 2% soln	60 to 75 min.	1	
With epinephrine		Soln, 1–2%	25 ml of 2% soln	2 hrs.	2	
mepivacaine	Carbocaine	Soln, 1–2%	15 ml of 2% soln	2 to 3 hrs	4	Amide
procaine	Novocaine	Soln, 1–4%	38 ml of 2% soln	30 to 45 min.	3	Ester

(3) Adjuncts$^\psi$

Drug	Trade	Preparation	Usual Dose	Notes
hyaluronidase	Vitrase	200 USP units/ml	50–300 units, typical dose 150 USP units	Depolymerizes polysaccharides and increases effective area of anesthesia, decreases duration of local anesthesia
		Lyophilized, 6200 USP units	Reconstitute to 1000 USP units/vial by adding 6.2 ml of solution to the vial. Common dose is 150 USP units	Depolymerizes polysaccharides and increases effective area of anesthesia, decreases duration of local anesthesia
sodium bicarbonate		1 mEq/ml	1 ml in 10 ml anesthetic	Decreases pain on injection

(4) Intraocular$^{\psi}$

Drug	Trade	Preparation	Usual Dose	Notes
lidocaine	Xylocaine	1%, non-preserved , without epinephrine	0.5 ml	**Intraocular** adjunct for cataract surgery do with "topical anesthesia"

Note: Intraocular bupivacaine may be harmful to the corneal endothelium and should be avoided for intraocular cases (Am J Ophthalmol 1999;127:393–402)

$^{\psi}$ Data taken from Ophthalmology Monograph 8, *Surgery of the Eyelid, Orbit, and Lacrimal System,* American Academy of Ophthalmology, 1993

^{x}1 = least painful, 5 = most painful

$^{\infty}$Allergic cross-reactions between groups do not occur. If patient allergic to ester compounds, amides may tried

F. HOMEOPATHIC DRUGS

Note: The authors do not generally prescribe these remedies; however, the information is provided below.

Drug	Trade	Preparation	Usual Dose	Notes
N/A	Optique	Soln	PRN	preservative-free homeopathic drug for eye irritation from allergy, fatigue, & pollution
N/A	Simalasan #1	Soln	5–6 × day PRN	homeopathic drug for dry eyes, preserved with Solusept
N/A	Simalasan #2	Soln	5–6 × day PRN	homeopathic drug for allergic conjunctivitis, preserved with Solusept
succus cinarium maritima	SCM	Soln	BID	homeopathic drug marketed to retard progression of cataracts

G. CAPSULE STAINING ADJUNCTS

Drug	Trade	Preparation	Usual Dose	Notes
indocyanine green	IC-Green	see notes	0.5 ml intraocular	may be used as an adjunct to stain the anterior capsule for **cataract surgery**; preparation involves adding 0.5 cc of the aqueous solvent into the power vial. After shaking, dilute this with 4.5 cc of balanced salt solution to bring total volume to 5 cc (Arch Ophthalmol 1998;116:535–537). Must be used within 10 hours of mixing. Should be avoided in patients with a history of allergy to iodine containing products
trypan blue	Vision Blue	Soln, 0.06%	0.5 ml intraocular	used as an adjunct to stain the anterior capsule for **cataract surgery**; does not require reconstitution; caution – may stain hydrophilic acrylic intraocular lenses or other structures within the eye such as the anterior vitreous face

H. MISCELLANEOUS

Drug	Trade	Preparation	Usual Dose	Notes
acetylcysteine	Mucomyst	Soln, 10%, 20%	QID	for **filamentary keratopathy**
alteplase	Activase	intra-ocular	6.25–12.5 micrograms/day	for clot dissolution post-vitrectomy
disodiumEDTA	Endrate	Soln, 15%	applied by physician	for **band keratopathy** used as a 3% solution, diluted from the 15% solution
				do **not** use dicalcium EDTA
cysteamine		Soln, 0.5%	Q 1 hr while awake	for **cystinosis** corneal crystals (Arch. Ophthalmol 1990. Vol 108 p.689)
dapsone		tabs, 25 & 100 mg	25–200 mg PO BID	for **ocular cicatricial pemphigoid**° must exclude G6PD deficiency and monitor reticulocyte count, hemoglobin/hematocrit to monitor for hemolytic anemia
povidone-iodine	Betadine Sterile Ophthalmic Prep Solution	Soln, 5%	applied as part of pre-operative preparation	part of sterile prep for operative procedures
silver nitrate		Soln, 1% (in wax ampules)	applied by physician	for **superior limbic keratoconjunctivitis**°; do **not** use sticks or higher concentration solutions
tyloxapol	Enuclene	Soln, 0.25%	TID-QID PRN	cleaning/lubricating solution for artificial eyes
white petrolatum/ mineral oil/ steric acid	Stye Ophthalmic Ointment	Oint, 55%/32%	PRN	for external use only, **not** for ocular use. Marketed to relieve some of the symptoms associated with a **hordeolum**

° Refer to Wills Eye Manual: Office and Emergency Room Diagnosis and Treatment of Eye Disease for protocol

I. DRUGS FOR HYPHEMA

Drug	Trade	Preparation	Usual Dose	Notes
aminocaproic acid	Amicar	syrup, 250 mg/ml tabs, 500 mg	50 mg/kg PO Q 4 hrs. (max dose = 30 Gm/day)	for **hyphema**[fz] orthostatic hypotension is significant side effect
	Carbopol	30% aminocaproic acid in 2% carboxypolymethylene gel	Q 6 hrs	Topical therapy for **hyphema**[k]
tranexamic acid			75 mg/kg/day in 3 divided doses for 5 days	alternative therapy for traumatic **hyphema** (Ophthalmology 1999;106:375–9)

[f] Ophthalmol 1998. 105;1715–1720
[k] Arch Ophthalmol 1997. 115;1106–1112
[z] Not for pregnant women or patients with renal failure, coagulopathy

11. Anti-Angiogenesis Agents

D.J. Rhee et al., *Ophthalmologic Drug Guide*, 2nd ed.,
DOI 10.1007/978-1-4419-7621-5_11,
© Springer Science+Business Media, LLC 2011

Drug	Trade	Preparation	Usual Dose	Notes
verteporfin	Visudyne	Soln, 2 mg/ml (supplied as 15 mg of lyophilized powder to be diluted in 7.5 ml of sterile water)	See appendix 7	For **photodynamic therapy** for subfoveal **choroidal neovascularization**
pegaptanib sodium	Macugen	0.3 mg intravitreal Q6 weeks		(N Engl J Med 2004; 351: 2805–16.) **Note:** Approved by the FDA for all subtypes (predominantly classic, minimally classic, occult) of CNV secondary to age-related macular degeneration (AMD)
ranibizumab	Lucentis	0.5 mg intravitreal Qmonth		Approved for the treatment of all subtypes of CNV secondary to AMD and for treatment of macular edema secondary to BRVO and CRVO
bevacizumab	Avastin	1.25 mg intravitreal		Intravitreal injection of bevacizumab is an off-label use of the drug. We do not yet have results of the randomized clinical trial of its use for AMD at the time of the writing of this book but it is widely used for this indication. It is also widely used for macular edema of various etiologies and retinal and iris neovascularization
triamcinolone acetate	Kenalog Triesence	4.0 mg intravitreal 20–40 mg sub-Tenon's		Intravitreal injection of triamcinolone acetate has been used in the treatment of macular edema of various etiologies and for uveitis

12. Contact Lens Solutions

D.J. Rhee et al., *Ophthalmologic Drug Guide*, 2nd ed.,
DOI 10.1007/978-1-4419-7621-5_12,
© Springer Science+Business Media, LLC 2011

Identifying the best system for a patient involves evaluation of patient's needs, the type of lenses worn, allergies, solution sensitivities, and the lens replacement schedule. The efficacy of lens care systems has been carefully evaluated by the manufacturers and approved by the FDA as safe and effective. These systems are tested (and proven efficacious) when used all together (i.e. as a "system" not each isolated product).

Contact Lens Solution Hypersensitivity

In any patients which sensitivities to ingredients are a strong possibility, the use of preservative-free care systems is strongly recommended. ALL products need to be switched to non-preserved, whenever these lenses are exposed to products that the patient is sensitive to, the lenses usually need to be replaced in order to solve any related problems. This is not typically true of rigid lenses (since they are not hydrophilic, they do not absorb the solution).

Soft Contact Lens Solutions

The products are listed in two ways – in the first section, all products are listed and divided by the type of lens care product. The categories of lens care products available are as follows:

– Daily Cleaner
– Saline Solution
– Disinfecting Solution
– Enzymatic Cleaners/Daily Protein Remover
– Multipurpose (all-in-one) Solutions
– Rewetting/Lubricating Drops

As a general rule, lens care regimens take into consideration the lens replacement schedule:

Conventional lenses – require the use of a daily cleaner (on a daily basis), daily disinfection, and weekly enzymatic cleaning. Replacement of these lenses is usually at least once a year (minimum).

Frequent or planned replacement lenses – (lenses replaced monthly, bimonthly, or quarterly) also require daily cleaning, daily disinfection, and weekly enzymatic cleaning.

Disposable lenses – (lenses replaced at least every two weeks) Daily cleaning is strongly recommended. Daily disinfection is absolutely necessary. Multipurpose solutions are most commonly used and recommended for these lenses and lens wearing modality.

Single Use lenses – Should never be reused. Therefore, do not need any care system. The only product suggested with these lenses is lubricating drops

Data compiled from Tylers Quarterly Soft Contac Lens Parameter Guide 2005, volume 22, No. 4 and manufacturer's package inserts

I. LISTING OF SOFT LENS PRODUCTS BY CATEGORY

A. Daily Cleaners

Product Name	Preservative	Notes
LENS PLUS® Daily Cleaner	Preservative Free	Not for direct use in eye
MiraFlow® Extra-Strength Cleaner	Isopropyl Alcohol	
Opti-Clean II	Polyquad	Not for direct use in eye
Opti-Free® Daily Cleaner	Polyquad	Not for direct use in eye
Pliagel® Cleaning Solution	Sorbic Acid	Not for direct use in eye
Sof/Pro Clean SA	Sorbic Acid and Edetate trisodium 0.25%	Not for direct use in eye

B. Enzymatic Cleaners

Name	Preservative	Active Ingredient	Warnings
COMPLETE® moisture Plus Weekly Enzymatic Cleaner	Tablet form – no preservative	Subtilisin A	Manufacturer recommends only using with other products from the Complete brand
Opti-Free® Enzymatic Cleaner Especially for Sensitive Eyes	Preservative Free	Pancreatin (for papain sensitive patients)	
Opti-Zyme® Enzymatic Cleaner Especially for Sensitive Eyes	Preservative Free	Pancreatin	Do Not Dissolve in Distilled Water
ReNu® One Step Enzymatic Cleaner	Tablet form – no preservative	Subtilisin A	Dissolve tablets only in ReNu Multipurpose Solution
ULTRAZYME® Enzymatic Cleaner	Tablet form – no preservative	Subtilisin A	
UNIZYME ENZYMATIC CLEANER	Tablet form – no preservative	Subtilisin A	For use with AOSEPT Pure Eyes, Quick-Care and Solo-Care disinfection systems.

C. Daily Protein Removers

Product Name	Preservative	Notes
CLERZ PLUS Lens Drops		Not for use directly in eye
RENU Liquid Enzymatic Cleaner	Contains Substilin A	Not for use directly in eye

D. Rewetting/Lubricating Drops

Product Name	Preservative	Notes
Aquify Long Lasting Comfort Drops	Sodium perborate	
Blink Contacts	Ocupure (stabilized oxychloro complex) 0.005%	
CIBA Vision® Lens Drops	Edetate Disodium 0.2% and Sorbic Acid 0.15%	
Clerz® 2 Lubricating and Rewetting Drops	Edetate Disodium and Sorbic Acid	
Clerz® PLUS Lens Drops	Edetate Disodium and Polyquad 0.001%	
COMPLETE® Blink-N-Clean Lens Drops	Polyhexamethylene Biguanide 0.0001%	
COMPLETE® moisture Plus Lubricating and Rewetting Drops	Polyhexamethylene Biguanide 0.0001%	
FOCUS LENS DROPS	Sorbic acid 0.15% and Edetate disodium 0.2%	
LENS COMFORT LENS LUBRICANT	Unknown	
LENS PLUS® Rewetting Drops	Preservative Free	
Opti-Free® EXPRESSRewetting Drops	Polyquad 0.001%	
Opti-One® Rewetting Drops	Polyquad 0.001%	Not for use directly in eye
Refresh Contacts	Preservative Free	
Refresh Contacts	0.005% Purite	
ReNu® MultiPlus ™ Lubricating and Rewetting drops	Edetate Disodium	
ReNu® Rewetting Drops	Edetate Disodium 0.1% and Sorbic Acid 0.15%	
Sensitive Eyes® Drops	Edetate Disodium 0.025% and Sorbic Acid 0.1%	
THERATEARS Contact Lens Comfort Drops	Sodium perborate	
VIVA-DROPS	Edetate Disodium 0.1% and Sorbic acid 0.25%	

E. Oxidation Solutions/Systems

Product Name	Preservative	Notes
AOSEPT® Clear Care Cleaning and Disinfection Solution	Hydrogen Peroxide 3% System	Requires neutralizing
AOSEPT® Disinfection/Neuralization Solution	Hydrogen Peroxide 3% System	Requires neutralizing
PureEyes™ Disinfection/Soaking Solution	Hydrogen Peroxide 3% System	Requires neutralizing
PureEyes™ Cleaner/Rinse		To be used with PureEyes™ Disinfection/Soaking Solution
ULTRACARE® Disinfecting Solution/Neutralizer Solution	Hydrogen Peroxide 3% system	Requires neutralizing

F. Saline Solutions

Product name	Preservative	Notes
Sterile Saline Solution	Preservative Free (aersol can)	made by Blairex Labs
Good Sense Saline Solution	Sorbic acid 0.1 % edentate disodium	
LENS PLUS® Sterile Saline Solution	Preservative Free	
Saline Solution Especially for Sensitive Eyes	Sorbic acid 0.125% and edentate disodium 0.1%	
Sensitive Eyes® Plus	DYMED and EDTA	
Sensitive Eyes® Saline Solution	Sorbic Acid 0.1% and Edetate Disodium 0.025%	
SoftWear® Saline	Sodium perborate turns into hydrogen peroxide	
Unisol® 4 Preservative Free Saline Solution	Preservative Free	

G. Combination Solutions

Name	Preservative	Notes
Aquify MPS	Polyhexanide 0.0001%	
Clear Conscience Mulipurpose Solution	Polyhexamethylene biguanide 0.001%	
Equate Multipurpose Solution	Polyhexamethylene biguanide 0.001%	
Opti-Free® Express™ MPDS Lasting Comfort No Rub Formula	Polyquad 0.001%	contains ALDOX™ – marketed as an anti-microbial to have cidal activity against both Acanthamoeba cysts and fungi
Opti-Free Rising, Disinfection and Storage Solutuion	Polyquad 0.001%	
Opti-ONE® Multi-Purpose Solution	Polyquad 0.001%	Tetronic and Pantionic removes protein
Quick-Care 5-Minute Cleaning and Disinfection System	Trace amounts of hydrogen peroxide	
ReNu® Multi-Purpose Solution	DYMED™ and Edetate Disodium	
ReNu with Moisture loc Multi-Purpose Solution	Alexidine	
ReNu Muli-Purpose Solution – NO RUB Solution	DYMED and Edetate disocium (no enzymatic cleaner needed)	
Sauflon Lite No Rub Multipurpose solution	Unknown	

II. SOFT LENS PRODUCTS LISTED BY SYSTEM AND MANUFACTURER: NOT ALL PRODUCTS ARE LISTED IN THIS SECTION BECAUSE NOT ALL PRODUCTS BELONG TO A PARTICULAR SYSTEM

Disinfection	Rinsing	Surfactant/Cleaning Agent	Wetting Solution	Enzymatic Cleaner
Opti-Free – Alcon				
Opti-Free® Express ™ MPDS	Opti-Free® Express ™ MPDS	Opti-Free® Express ™ MPDS	Clerz Plus Lens Drops **OR** Opti-Free Express Rewetting Drops	None needed
Opti-One Muli-Purpose Solution	Opti-One Muli-Purpose Solution	Opti-One Muli-Purpose Solution	Clerz Plus Lens Drops	Opti-Free Supraclens Daily Protein Remover
Opti-Free® Rinsing Disinfecting and Storage Solution	Opti-Free® Rinsing Disinfecting and Storage Solution	Opti-Free® Daily Cleaner	Clerz Plus Lens Drops	Opti-Free Supraclens Daily Protein Remover
ReNu – Bausch and Lomb				
ReNu® Plus Multi-Purpose Solution	ReNu® Plus Multi-Purpose Solution	ReNu® Plus Multi-Purpose Solution	ReNu Rewetting Drops	ReNu One-Step Enzymatic Cleaner
ReNu® Plus Multi-Purpose Solution No Rub Formula	ReNu® Plus Multi-Purpose Solution No Rub Formula	ReNu® Plus Multi-Purpose Solution No Rub Formula	ReNu Rewetting Drops	None needed

AOSEPT – CIBA

AOSEPT® Clear Care Cleaning and Disinfection Solution	Not Applicable	AOSEPT® Clear Care Cleaning and Disinfection Solution	CIBA Vision Lens Drops	Any non-thermal enzymatic cleaner
AOSEPT® Disinfecttion/Neutralizing Solution	SoftWear Saline	CIBA Vision Vision Cleaner OR MiraFlow Cleaner	CIBA Vision Lens Drops	Any non-thermal enzymatic cleaner
Pure Eyes Disinfectant/Soaking Solution	Pure Eyes Cleaner/Rinse	Pure Eyes Cleaner/Rinse	CIBA Vision Lens Drops	Any non-thermal enzymatic cleaner
Quick Care 5-minte Starting Solution	Quick Care 5-minte Finishing Solution	Quick Care 5-minte Starting Solution	CIBA Vision Lens Drops	Any non-thermal enzymatic cleaner

Advanced Medical Optics, Inc

Complete Moisture Plus Multi-Purpose Solution	Complete Moisture Plus Multi-Purpose Solution	Complete Moisture Plus Multi-Purpose Solution	Complete Moisture Plus Lubriation/Rewetting Drops OR Complete Blink-N-Clean	Complete Moisture Plus Weekly Enzymatic Cleaner
Ultracare Disinfection/Neutralizing Solution	Lens Plus Aerosol Saline	Lens Plus Daily Cleaner	Lens Plus Rewetting Drops OR Complete Blink-N-Clean	Ultrazyme Enzymatic Cleaner

Rigid Lens Solutions

As with soft lens care systems, rigid lens care systems are most effective when used as a "system," avoiding mixing and matching of products from different systems. Rigid lenses must be cleaned daily (with a daily cleaner) and disinfected daily (soaking in a disinfecting solution over night). Weekly enzymatic cleaning is also recommended.

The products are listed in two ways – in the first section, all products are listed and divided by the type of lens care product. The categories of lens care products available are as follows:

– Daily Cleaner
– Saline Solution
– Enzymatic Cleaners
– Daily Protein Removers
– Cleaning/Soaking/Disinfecting Solutions/Multipurpose (all-in-one) Solutions
– Laboratory Cleaners (polishing/cleaning compounds)

I. LISTING OF RIGID LENS RODUCTS BY CATEGORY

A. Daily Cleaners

Name	Preservative	Notes
BOSTON Advance® Cleaner	Preservative Free	Not for direct use in eye
BOSTON® Cleaner	Preservative Free	Not for direct use in eye
Claris Cleaning and Soaking Solution	Unknown	
Concentrated Cleaner	Unknown	
Non-Allergenic Clear Clean	Sorbic Acid	made by Contex – sold only to practitioners
Opti-Clean II®	Polyquad	Not for direct use in eye; approved for PMMA lenses only

	Preservative	Active Ingredients	Notes
Optimum by Lobob Extra Strength Cleaner	Unknonwn		
Perma-Brite	Not available		made by Danker Laboratories Inc.
Polish Brite/Super Cleaner Non-Allergenic	Sorbic Acid		made by Contex-sold only to practitioners
RESOLVE/GP® Daily Cleaner	Preservative Free		Not for direct use in eye
Sereine™ Cleaner	Edetate Disodium 0.1%, and Benzalkonium Chloride 0.01%		Not for direct use in eye
Serine Soaking and Cleaning	Unknown		Not for direct use in eye

B. Enzymatic Cleaners

Name	Preservative	Active Ingredients	Notes
Boston® One Step Liquid Enzymatic Cleaner	Preservative Free	Subtilisin	
PROFREE/GP® Weekly Enzymatic Cleaner	Edetate Disodium	Papain	Not to be dissolved in distilled water

C. Daily Protein Remover

Name	Preservative	Notes
Opti-Free® Supraclens® Daily Protein Remover	Preservative Free	Not for direct use in the eye

D. Oxidation Systems

Name	Preservative	Notes
AOSEPT Clear Care Cleaning and Disinfection Solution	3% Hydrogen Peroxide	

E. Storage and Disinfection

Name	Preservative	Notes
BOSTON Advance® Comfort Formula Conditioning Solution	Edetate Disodium 0.05%, Polyaminopropyl Biguanide 0.0005%, Chlorhexidine Gluconate 0.003%	
BOSTON® Conditioning Solution	Edetate Disodium 0.05%, Chlorhexidine Gluconate 0.006%	
Barnes-Hind ComfortCare® GP Wetting and Soaking Solution	Edetate Disodium 0.02% and Chlorhexidine Gluconate 0.005%	
Claris Cleaning and Soaking Solution	Benzyl Alcohol 0.39% and Trisodium Edetate 0.5%	Not for direct use in eye
Sereine™ Wetting and Soaking Solution	Edetate Disodium 0.1% and Benzalkonium Chloride 0.01%	
WET-N-SOAK PLUS®	Edetate Disodium and Benzalkonium Chloride 0.003%	
Wetting and Soaking Solution		Bausch and Lomb

F. Wetting/Rewetting

Name	Preservative	Notes
AQuify Long Lasting Comfort Drops	Not Available	
Blink contacts	Not Available	
CIBA Vision Lens Drops	Not Available	
Clerz Plus Lens Drops	Not Available	
Complete Blink-N-Clean Lens Drops	Not Available	
BOSTON® Rewetting Drops	Edetate Disodium 0.05% and Chlorhexadine Gluconate 0.006%	
CLARIS™ Rewetting Drops	Hydroxyethyl Cellulose, Polixetonium Chlorine 0.006%	
Optimum by Lobob Wetting and Rewetting Drops	Edetate Disodium, Sorbic Acid, Benzyl Alcohol	
Perma-Cote	Benzalkonium Chloride 0.002%	
Sereine™ Wetting Solution	Edetate Disodium 0.1% and Benzalkonium Chloride 0.01%	
TheraTears Contact Lens Comfort Drops	Not Available	

G. Combination Solutions

Name	Preservative	Notes
BOSTON Simplicity® Multi-Action Solution	Edetate Disodium 0.05%, Polyaminopropyl Biguanide 0.0005%, Chlorhexadine Gluconate 0.003%	
BOSTON Simplus Multi-Action Solution	Not Available	
Lens Comfort Multipurpose Solution	Not Available	
Optimum by Lobob C/D/S	Not Available	
Unique-pH Multi-Purpose Solution	Not Available	

APPENDIX 1: TOPICAL ANTIBACTERIAL SPECTRUM

Legend:
+ = sensitive
o = not sensitive
i = intermediate activity

FR = fluoroquinolone resistant

baci = bacitracin
CAM = chloramphenicol
cipro = ciprofloxacin
ceph = cephazolin
erythro = erythromycin

gati = gatifloxacin
gent = gentamicin
levo = levofloxacin
norflox = norfloxacin
moxi = moxifloxacin

oflox = ofloxacin
poly/trimeth = polymyxin B/trimethoprim
sulfa = sulfacetamide
tetra/poly = tetracycline/polymyxin B
tobra = tobramycin
vanco = vancomycin

	baci	cephazolin	CAM	cipro	erythro	gati	gent	levo	moxi	norflox	oflox	polymyxin B	poly/ trimeth	sulfa	tetra/ poly	tobra	vanco
Staph aureus (MS)	+	+	+	+	i	?	+	+	?	+	+	o	+	+	+	+	+
Staph aureus FR	?	?	?	–	?	–	–	–	+	–	–	?	?	?	?	?	?
Staph epidermadis	+	i	o	+	o	+	+	+	+	+	+	o	+	o	+	+	+
Staph coag neg FR	?	?	?	–	?	i	–	–	i	–	–	?	?	?	?	?	?
Strep pyogenes	+	+	o	+	+	+	+	+	+	o	+	o	+	o	+	+	+
Strep pneumo	+	+	+	+	+	+	+	+	+	+	I	o	+	+	+	+	+
Strep viridans	+	+	+	+	+	+	+	+	+	o	I	o	+	+	+	+	+
Enterococcus faecalis	+	o	o	i	o	?	+	?	?	+	+	o	+	o	o	o	+
Bacillus cereus	o	o	+	+	+	?	+	?	?	+	?	o	o	o	i	+	+
E. coli	o	+	+	+	o	+	+	+	+	+	+	+	+	+	+	+	o
H. influenzea	o	+	+	+	i	+	+	+	+	+	+	o	+	+	+	+	o
Klebsiella	o	+	+	–	o	+	+	+	+	+	I	+	+	+	+	+	o

(continued)

D.J. Rhee et al., *Ophthalmologic Drug Guide*, 2nd ed.,
DOI 10.1007/978-1-4419-7621-5,
© Springer Science+Business Media, LLC 2011

APPENDIX 1: TOPICAL ANTIBACTERIAL SPECTRUM (continued)

	baci	cephazolin	CAM	cipro	erythro	gati	gent	levo	moxi	norflox	oflox	polymyxin B	poly/trimeth	sulfa	tetra/poly	tobra	vanco
Enterobacter	0	0	+	+	0	+	+	+	+	+	+	+	+	+	0	+	0
Moraxella species	0	+	+	+	0	+	+	+	0	0	+	0	0	0	0	0	0
Neisseria species	+	+	+	+	+	+	+	+	+	+	+	0	0	0	0	+	i
Pseud. aeruginosa	0	0	+	+	0	+	+	+	0	0	+	i	i	i	+	+	0
Pseud aeruginosa FR	?	?	?	–	?	–	–	–	–	–	–	?	?	?	?	?	?
Serratia marcescens	0	0	+	+	0	+	+	+	0	0	+	0	+	0	0	+	0
Aeromonas	0	0	i	+	0	+	+	+	+	+	+	0	0	0	0	0	0
Acinetobacter	+	0	0	+	0	+	+	+	+	+	+	i	0	0	0	+	0
Bacteroides fragilis	0	0	+	0	0	+	0	+	0	0	+	0	0	0	0	0	0
Proprionobacter acnes	0	0	0	i	i	0	0	0	0	0	0	0	0	0	i	0	+

Table compiled from information from *Physicians Desk Reference for Ophthalmology.* 1999. *Sanford Guide to Antimicrobial Therapy,* 1995. Sanford, JP., Gilbert, DN., Sande, MA., and *Goodman and Gilman's The Pharmacological Basis of Therapeutics.* 1990. Gilman, AG., Rall, TW., Nies, AS., Taylor, P. 8th Ed. Pergamon Press, and *Manual of Clinical Microbiology.* 1995. Murray, PR., Baron, EJ., Pfaller, MA., Tenover, FC., Yolken, RH. 6th Ed. ASM Press. 1995. Graves A, et al. Cornea 2001;3:301–305. Kowalski RP., et al Am J Ophthalmol 2003;136:500–505. Hwang DG. Surv Ophthalmol 2004;49:S79–S83. Mather R, et al. Am J Ophthalmol 2002;133:463–466. Fiscella RG, et al Ophthalmology 1999;106:2286–2290

APPENDIX 2: A PREPARING FORTIFIED TOPICAL ANTIBIOTICS AND PREPARING ORAL ACETAZOLAMIDE SOLUTION

Fortified Bacitracin

Add enough sterile water (without preservative) to 50,000 U of bacitracin dry powder to form 5 mL of solution. This provides a strength of 10,000 U/mL. Refrigerate. Expires after 7 days.

Fortified Cefazolin

Add enough sterile water (without preservative) to 500 mg of cefazolin dry powder to form 10 mL of solution. This provides a strength of 50 mg/mL. Refrigerate. Expires after 7 days.

Fortified Tobramycin (or Gentamicin)

With a syringe, inject 2 mL of tobramycin 40 mg/mL directly into a 5 mL bottle of tobramycin 0.3% ophthalmic solution (e.g., Tobrex). This gives a 7 mL solution of fortified tobramycin (approximately 15 mg/mL). Refrigerate. Expires after 14 days.

Fortified Vancomycin

Add enough sterile water (without preservative) to 500 mg of vancomycin dry powder to form 10 mL of solution. This provides

a strength of 50 mg/mL. To achieve a 25 mg/mL concentration, take 5 mL of 50 mg/mL solution and add 5 mL sterile water. Refrigerate. Expires after 4 days.

Reference:

Rhee DJ, Pyfer MF, eds. The Wills Eye Manual. Philadelphia: J. B. Lippincott, 1999, p. 520.

Dilute IV preparation in fruit juice such that one teaspoon (5 cc) contains correct unit dose (5–10 mg/kg/dose) (expensive) or prepare suspension with crushed pills and shake well. Expires after 5 days.

Add contents of one 500 mg IV vial to 500 ml fruit juice – shake well to dispurse. This gives a 5 mg/5 ml (teaspoonful). Must shake well before using.

APPENDIX 3: ANTI-FUNGAL ACTIVITY SPECTRUM

Notes:
1) Candida develops resistance quickly to flucytosine
2) Information compiled from information from *Physicians Desk Reference* (1999)
3) Table represents in-vitro sensitivites which may or may not correlate with in-vivo situations. Additionally, sensitivites will vary among institutions.

	Aspergillus	Blastomyces	Candida	Coccidiodes	Cryptococcus	Fusarium	Histoplasma	Penicillium	Z. Mucor
Amphotericin	X	X	X	X	X	X/–	X	X/–	X
Fluconazole	O	O	X	O	X	O	O	O	O
Flucytosine	O	O	X	O	X	O	O	O	O
Itraconazole	O	X	X	O	X/–	O	X	O	O
Ketoconazole	O	O	X	O	O	O	X	O	O
Miconazole	X	O	X	O	X	O	O	O	O
Natamycin	X	O	X	O	O	X	O	X	O

APPENDIX 4: RENAL DOSING FOR SELECTED DRUGS

Dosing in Renal Impairment (adjust creatinine clearance for body surface area)*

Oral

Normal dosage regimen	Creatinine clearance (mL/min/1.73 m²)	Adjusted dosage regimen Dose (mg)	Dosing interval
200 mg q4 hours (5×/day)	>10	200	q4 hours (5×/day)
	0–10	200	q12 hours
400 mg q12 hours	>10	400	q12 hours
	0–10	200	q12 hours
800 mg q4 hours (5×/day)	>25	800	q4 hours (5×/day)
	10–25	800	q8 hours
	0–10	800	q12 hours

Intravenous

Creatinine Clearance (mL/min/1.73 m²)	Percent of recommended dose	Dosing interval
>50	100 %	q8 hours
25–50	100 %	q12 hours
10–25	100 %	q24 hours
0–10	50 %	q24 hours

Cidofovir Dosing in Renal Failure[*]

Dose must be reduced from 5 mg/kg to 3 mg/kg for an increase in creatinine of 0.3–0.4 mg/dl above baseline
Discontinue for increase ≥ 0.5 mg/kg above baseline or development of ≥ 3+ proteinuria

Famciclovir Dosing in Renal Failure[*]

Creatinine clearance (mL/min)	adjusted dose
>60	500 mg every 8 hours
40–59	500 mg every 12 hours
20–39	500 mg every 24 hours
<20	250 mg every 24 hours
hemodialysis	250 mg following each dialysis

Foscarnet Dosing in Renal Failure[*]

Creatinine Clearance (ml/min)	Resistant HSV (mg/kg)	CMV Induction (mg/kg)
> 1.4	40 Q12 hrs	40 Q8 hrs
> 1.0–1.4	30 Q12 hrs	30 Q8 hrs
> 0.8–1.0	20 Q12 hrs	35 Q12 hrs
> 0.6–0.8	35 Q24 hrs	25 Q12 hrs
> 0.5–0.6	25 Q24 hrs	40 Q24 hrs
≥ 0.4–0.5	20 Q24 hrs	35 Q24 hrs
< 0.4	Not Recommended	Not Recommended

Creatinine Clearance (ml/min)	CMV maintenance [equiv. to 60 mg/kg Q8 hrs]	CMV maintenance [equiv. to 90 mg/kg Q8 hrs]
> 1.4	60 Q8 hrs	90 Q12 hrs
> 1.0–1.4	45 Q8 hrs	70 Q12 hrs
> 0.8–1.0	50 Q12 hrs	50 Q12 hrs
> 0.6–0.8	40 Q12 hrs	80 Q24 hrs
> 0.5–0.6	60 Q24 hrs	60 Q24 hrs
≥ 0.4–0.5	50 Q24 hrs	50 Q24 hrs
< 0.4	Not Recommended	Not Recommended

Creatinine Clearance (ml/min)	CMV maintenance (mg/kg) [equiv. to 90 mg/kg/day]	[equiv. to 120 mg/kg/day]
>1.4	90 q24 hrs	120 q24 hrs
>1.0–1.4	70 q24 hrs	90 q24 hrs
>0.8–1.0	50 q24 hrs	65 q24 hrs
>0.6–0.8	80 q48 hrs	105 q48 hrs
>0.5–0.6	60 q48 hrs	80 q48 hrs
≥0.4–0.5	50 q48 hrs	65 q48 hrs
<0.4	Not recommended	Not recommended

Intravenous Ganciclovir Dosing in Renal Failure*

Creatinine clearance (ml/min)	Induction dose (mg/kg)	Dosing interval (hours)	Maintenance dose (mg/kg)	Dosing interval (hours)
≥ 70	5.0	12	5.0	24
50–69	2.5	12	2.5	24
25–49	2.5	24	1.25	24
10–24	1.25	24	0.625	24
< 10	1.25	3×/week after hemodialysis	0.625	3×/week after hemodialysis

Oral Ganciclovir Dosing in Renal Failure*

Creatinine clearance (ml/min)	Capsule dose
≥ 70	1000 mg tid or 500 mg q3 hrs, 6×/day
50–69	1500 mg qd or 500 mg tid
25–49	1000 mg qd or 500 mg bid
10–24	500 mg qd
< 10	500 mg 3×/week after hemodialysis

Valacyclovir Dosing in Renal Failure[*]

Creatinine clearance (mL/min)	adjusted dose
≥50	1 g po q8 hrs
30–49	1 g po q12 hrs
10–29	1 g po q24 hrs
<10	500 mg q24 hrs

[*] All tables taken from Physicians' Desk Reference, 1999
[*] All tables taken from Physicians' Desk Reference, 1997

Creatinine clearance for males: $\dfrac{(140 - \text{age[yrs]})\,(\text{body wt [kg]})}{(72)\,(\text{serum creatinine [mg/dL]})}$

Creatinine clearance for females: $0.85 \times$ male value

Note: Delete body weight from calculation for foscarnet since creatinine clearance units are different (ml/min/kg)

APPENDIX 5: GLAUCOMA MEDICATION PRESERVATIVES

There is a growing body of literature indicating that higher concentrations of BAK are associated with inflammatory changes in the conjunctiva and even trabecular meshwork.[1-2]

Preservative		Drug	Trade
None		timolol maleate	Timoptic (ocu-dose)
		pilocarpine 2% & 4%	generic (steri-unit)
Benzalkonium chloride	0.01%	apraclonidine	Iopidine
	0.01%	betaxolol	Betoptic
	0.005%	bimatoprost	Lumigan
	0.005%	brimonidine	Alphagan
	0.01%	brinzolamide	Azopt
		carbachol	Isopto Carbachol
	0.005%	carteolol	Carteolol HCl
		demecarium bromide	Humorsol
		dipivefrin	Propine
	0.0075%	dorzolamide	Trusopt
		epinephrine	Epifrin

Preservative	Concentration	Drug	Brand
	0.02%	latanoprost	Xalatan
	0.004%	levobunolol	Betagan
	0.004%	metipranolol	Optipranolol
		pilocarpine hydrochloride	Isopto Carpine, Pilocar, Pilostat, Pilopine HS gel
	0.01%	timolol maleate	Timoptic
	0.0075%	timolol maleate/dorzolamide	Cosopt
	0.01%	timolol hemihydrate	Betimol
	0.015%	travoprost	Travatan
	0.012%	timolol maleate	Timoptic XE
		echothiophate iodide	Phospholine Iodide
		pilocarpine nitrate	Pilagan
Benzododecinium bromide			
Chlorobutanol			
Purite (stabilized oxychloro complex)	0.005%	brimonidine 0.1%, 0.15%	Alphagan-P

1. Anwaruddin R, et al Invest Ophthalmol Vis Sci (Suppl) 2002;43:164
2. Baudouin C, et al Ophthalmology 1999;106:556–563

APPENDIX 6: TITRATING TOPICAL DROPS FOR CHILDREN

This table is given to help the clinician estimate how to adjust the adult eye drop dose for pediatric aged patients. Due to the infants smaller blood volume, systemic levels of topically applied drops can be very high compared to the adult. One study showed that infants using timolol maleate 0.25% had up to 25 times the adult plasma level (*Ophthalmology* 1984;91:1361–1363). Other considerations when attempting to limit systemic adsorption in children are:

1) Start with lower concentrations when therapeutically warrented and the alternative exists. (example timolol maleate 0.25% instead of 0.5%)

2) Use passive lid closure and digital pressure over the canalicular drainage system when possible to limit access to the nasal mucosa.

It is important to note that this table is not applicable to all children. Body weight, metabolic function, and concomitant medications should also be taken into account.

Age	Fraction of adult dose
birth–2 years old	50%
2–3 years old	67%
3–7 years old	90%
7–12 years old	95%
> 12 years old	full dose

Adapted from Abelson MB, Paradis A, Grant KK. How to prescribe for the smallest sufferers. *Review of Ophthalmology* 1999;2:101–103

APPENDIX 7: DOSING PROTOCOL FOR VERTEPORFIN (VISUDYNE)

Indication: Photodynamic therapy (PDT) for subfoveal choroidal neovascularization (CNV)

Supplied as: Comes as single use vial, 15 mg verteporfin, lyophilized. Reconstitute with 7 mL sterile water to provide 7.5 mL of 2 mg/mL.

Dose: 6 mg/m^2 diluted to 30 mL in 5% dextrose. Infusion is given over 10 minutes at a rate of 3 mL/minute using syringe pump and in-line filter.

Light administration: 689 nm wavelength of laser light exactly 15 minutes after the start of the 10 minute infusion (i.e. 5 minutes after the infusion ends). The exposure time is 83 seconds. [Recommended light dose is 50 J/cm^2 at an intensity of 600 mW/cm^2.]

Treatment: PDT is currently approved in the United States for the treatment of subfoveal predominantly classic CNV (> 50% classic) and subfoveal occult CNV with evidence of recent progression. Nasal edge of treatment spot must be at least 200 microns from the temporal edge of the optic disc, even if this will result in lack of treatment within 200 microns of the optic nerve. Spot size should be 1000 microns larger then greatest linear dimension of the CNV lesion. Maximum spot size used in clinical trials was 6400 microns.

Contraindicated in patients with porphyria

Treatment should be carefully considered in patients with moderate to severe hepatic impairment (eliminated via liver)

After dye administration, patients must avoid direct sunlight, indoor halogen lighting, tanning beds, or other bright lighting for 5 days.

Side effects: headache, injection site reaction, visual disturbance (including blurred vision, decreased vision, and visual field defects), and photosensitivity in 10–20% of patients

Other side effects occurring in < 10% of patients:

ocular: subretinal or vitreous hemorrhage

systemic: back pain (during infusion of dye), flu syndrome, elevated liver function tests, others

Product Index

Subject Index